BONE HEALTH BASICS

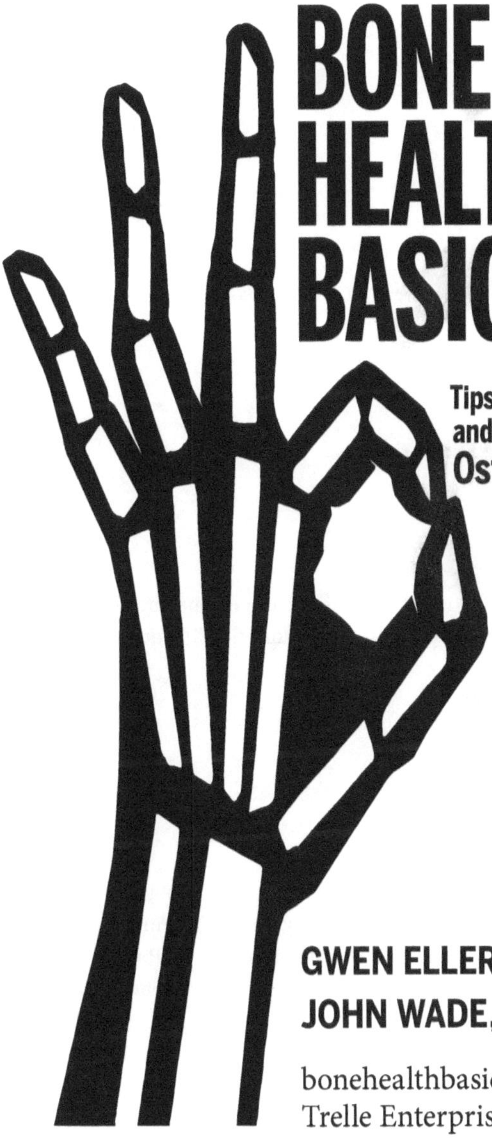

Tips for Preventing and Managing Osteoporosis

GWEN ELLERT, MEd, BScN

JOHN WADE, MD, FRCPC

bonehealthbasics.com
Trelle Enterprises Inc.

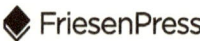 FriesenPress

Suite 300 - 990 Fort St
Victoria, BC, V8V 3K2
Canada

www.friesenpress.com

Copyright © 2020 by Trelle Enterprises Inc.
Vancouver, Canada
Tel 604-910-9694
First Edition — 2020

NOTICE: This text is not intended as a substitute for personal medical advice. Before taking any form of treatment, you should always consult with your physician.

Illustrations by Dave Hancock
Edited by Bruce Wells

bonehealthbasics.com

ISBN
978-1-5255-4811-6 (Hardcover)
978-1-5255-4812-3 (Paperback)
978-1-5255-4813-0 (eBook)

1. HEALTH & FITNESS, DISEASES, MUSCULOSKELETAL

Distributed to the trade by The Ingram Book Company

Contents

Foreword

We've all seen the headlines: "New drug reduces fractures by 70%." For many people, that's great news. Just take a pill and no more worrying about weak bones breaking.

Or, how about: "Calcium pills raise heart risk." Whoa! That's scary news. Many people take calcium supplements to maintain strong bones. Is it worth the risk if taking calcium pills leads to heart problems?

Lots of advertisements on television and in magazines we read tell us how this drug or that drug can help address a health problem or make us feel better. They tell us about potential side-effects and advise us to "be sure to talk to your doctor before taking any medication."

Of course, to clear up any misinformation or confusion, we ought to consult with our doctor or other healthcare professional. We can also search the internet for information. At the end of the day, however, it's up to us individually to determine which headlines we believe and, most importantly, decide which medications or supplements to take.

Most people will reach their peak bone mass before the age of 30 and will begin to lose bone mass by age 40. So, it is integral to build strong bones starting at an early age. The goal of this book is to help you better understand how your bones work, how to prevent bone loss, and how to prevent the first fracture from occurring and reduce the risk of future fractures. This book explains how your bones are affected when you have bone loss or osteoporosis. It teaches you about what is going on inside your body so you can ask the right questions and get the information you need in order to make relevant and timely decisions about your own bone health.

Bone Health Basics reviews risk factors for osteoporosis as well as for falls and fractures. We will introduce you to methods for self-managing your bone health and preventing fractures. We'll discuss the different treatment options for women and men who have low bone density or osteoporosis. You will discover how a calcium-rich diet, vitamin D and exercise can help you feel better so you can maintain the lifestyle you choose while living with less bone density or osteoporosis.

The content for this book is based on the fourth edition of *The Osteoporosis Book: Bone Health*, which provides more comprehensive information for patients and healthcare professionals (doctors, pharma-cists, nurses) on bone health and fracture prevention. *The Osteoporosis Book: Bone Health (Fourth Edition)* is available on Amazon.com

Osteoporosis is a major health problem and is increasingly common with age in both men and women, and with some diseases and medica-tions. Today's healthcare systems are moving toward patient-centered care. The goal of this type of care is to encourage patient empowerment through education and support from the healthcare team. By learning to under-stand how your bones work and what questions to ask about the issues that are important to your bone health, you will be able to take a more proactive role in your health and well-being.

Caring About Your Bone Health

You naturally build bone until your late teens or early twenties. After your mid-thirties you begin to lose more bone than you form.

By our mid-thirties we start to slowly lose bone. For women, bone loss occurs at a faster rate after menopause. As bone loss occurs, bones become weaker and more prone to breaking.

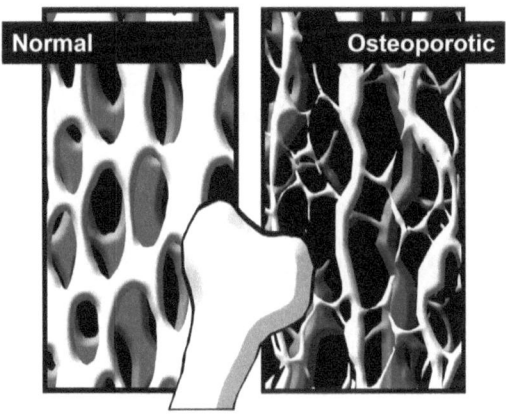

Osteoporosis can have a profound impact on a person's life. Osteoporosis and osteoporosis-related hip and spine fractures, for example, are linked to poorer quality of life and an increased risk of death. One-year post-hip fracture is associated with:

- *inability to carry out at least one independent activity of daily living*
- *inability to walk independently*
- *permanent disability or death*

If you have osteoporosis, you are at a higher risk of breaking a bone from a fall. The disease can also adversely affect your general state of health and well-being.

RISK FACTORS FOR OSTEOPOROSIS

FAMILY HISTORY OR GENETICS

- *age 50 or older*
- *parent had hip fracture*
- *low body weight or weight loss of more than 10% since age 25*
- *height loss of 1 inch (approximately 2 cm) in the last three years or more as measured by your healthcare provider, or 2.5 inches (approximately 6 cm) or more since your tallest known height*

LIFESTYLE

- *smoke tobacco products*
- *consume excessive amount of alcohol (three or more drinks/day)*
- *a woman who has excessive emotional or physical stress that disrupts or stops monthly periods*
- *diet low in calcium or vitamin D*
- *little exposure to sunlight, which may cause low vitamin D levels*
- *on extended bed rest*
- *inactive lifestyle, irregular or little physical activity*

MEDICAL HISTORY AND MEDICATIONS

- *diagnosed with rheumatoid arthritis*
- *diagnosed with celiac or other malabsorption disease*
- *diagnosed with chronic liver or kidney disease*
- *diabetes mellitus*
- *medications include antacids, anticoagulants, antidepressants, anticonvulsants*
- *history of glucocorticoid (prednisone) use*
- *estrogen/testosterone deficient*
- *prostate or breast cancer medication*
- *broke a bone after age 40 due to a low trauma fall or other mishap*
- *kidney, thyroid, parathyroid, ovarian or liver problems*
- *started menopause early (before age 45)*
- *eating disorders, such as anorexia nervosa, bulimia*

Sandy's Story: Low Bone Mass

Sandy, 42, is fit and active – regularly cycling, hiking, playing tennis and swimming. She eats a healthy diet complemented by some supplements and vitamins. She has never smoked, broken a bone or suffered from a significant disease.

Sandy recently participated in a research study on bone health in which she discovered she may have up to four times greater risk of fracture than the average 30-year-old female. For Sandy, this was a warning that she may be at risk of osteoporosis or fracture in the future.

ARE YOU AT RISK?

Take a minute to read this quick fracture risk assessment. The questions will give you an idea of what doctors look for when assessing your bone health.

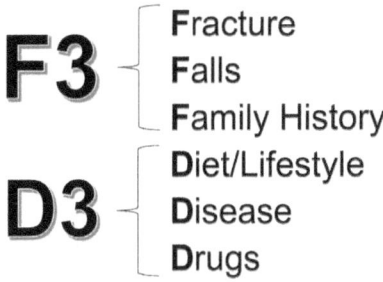

FRACTURE

- *Have you lost height, possibly indicating a vertebral (spinal) fracture?*
- *Have you had a non-vertebral fracture (e.g., of the wrist, hip, spine, shoulder) since age 40?*

FALLS

- *Have you fallen in the past year? If yes, how many times?*
- *If you are over 65 and have had more than one fall in the previous 12 months, you are at a high risk of fracture in the future.*

FAMILY HISTORY

- *Did either of your parents have osteoporosis or fracture a hip?*
- *Did either or your parents or grandparents have a stooped posture?*
- *Genetics may determine up to 80% of your risk for osteoporosis.*

DIET/LIFESTYLE

- *Is your daily diet consumption less than 1,200 mg of calcium or 800 IU of vitamin D?*
- *Are your arms and legs exposed to sunshine less than 10 mins/day?*
- *Do you regularly feel emotionally overstressed?*
- *Do you lack regular weight-bearing exercises (150 mins/week of moderate exercise or 30 mins/day five times a week)?*
- *Do you smoke?*
- *Do you drink alcohol more than the equivalent of three glasses of wine per day?*

DISEASE

- *Do you have a disease that puts you at risk of bone loss?*
- *Diseases that increase your risk of bone loss include celiac disease, alcoholism, rheumatoid arthritis.*

DRUGS

- *Do any of the medications you are taking increase your risk of bone loss? Check with your healthcare professional.*
- *Drugs that increase risk of bone loss include glucocorticoids, excess thyroid hormone, some ulcer medications.*
- *Drugs that increase risk of falling include sedatives, blood pressure medication, analgesics (pain medication).*

The good news is that for many people, the process of bone loss can be slowed down or reversed.

Proper nutrition, especially adequate intake of calcium and vitamin D, is important for bone health. During our younger years, we require a lot of calcium for bone formation. The dietary calcium we consume when we are young affects bone health for the rest of our lives. By building strong bones early, we will have more bone to draw upon as we age. If you did not get enough calcium when you were young and you are over 30, your focus should be on maintaining the bone you have. We will discuss more about building and maintaining bone in the next chapter.

Dietary intake is usually not enough to get adequate vitamin D. Exposure to the sun and supplementation is generally required. Routine daily supplementation of vitamin D is especially recommended for adults in colder climates whose skin does not receive much exposure to sunshine. You will find more information about vitamin D in Chapter 5.

Regular exercise can help to slow bone loss. Consider starting a walking program or a controlled weight training program that properly increases stress on the bone. Balance exercises to decrease falls are also helpful. Check with your healthcare professional before starting any exercise program. We will talk more about the importance of exercise in Chapter 6.

If you are at high risk of fracture, there are some medications your healthcare professional may prescribe. Later in the book we will discuss how to assess your bone health for fracture risk as well as some of the medications prescribed for preventing future fractures.

Read about Sandy's experience with low bone mass in Chapter 10.

What is Happening on the Inside

The goal is to prevent future fractures. Take precautions to reduce bone loss and prevent falls. Building high peak bone mass is important.

BONE DEVELOPMENT

- *Bone is a living tissue that is continually being formed and resorbed (removed).*
- *Normally, a child's bones grow because more bone is formed than resorbed.*
- *Bone loss for men and women begins in the mid-thirties.*
- *A greater-than-average imbalance in formation and resorption for your stage of life may lead to a problem with your bone strength (density and quality).*

BONE NOURISHMENT

- *Bone needs nutrients such as calcium, vitamin D and protein to develop and stay healthy.*
- *Hormones help to break down these nutrients and absorb them into the bloodstream and then bone tissue.*

FRACTURES

- *When a bone is stressed, it may fracture depending on the degree of its strength, density and amount of stress place on the bone.*
- *The most common areas of fracture with osteoporosis are the spine, hips and wrists.*

CAUSES OF OSTEOPOROSIS

- *Generally, osteoporosis can result from genetics, menopause, aging, immobility, endocrine (glandular) diseases and some medications.*

HOW THE BODY MOVES

To move easily, your bones should be strong enough to support your body weight. Your joints need to be flexible and your muscles need to be able to contract and relax.

The human skeleton consists of 206 separate bones. These bones provide:

- *the internal framework for the body, providing, among other things, support and protection for internal organs*
- *a point of attachment for muscles and tendons to support body movement*

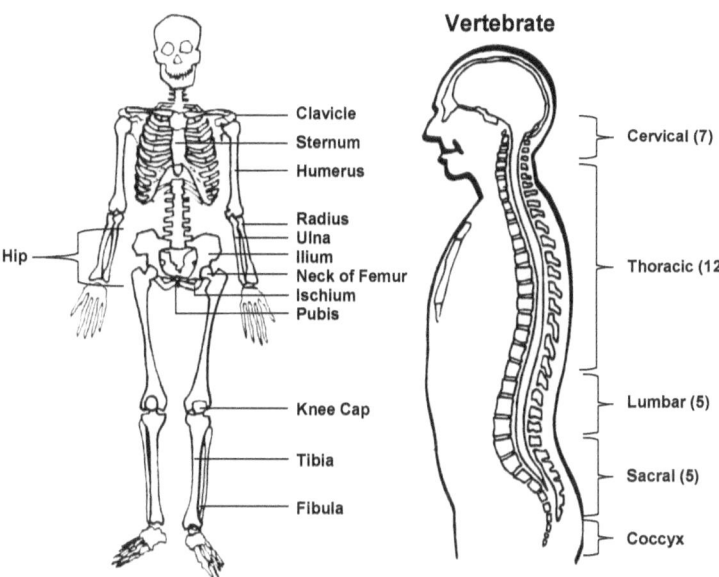

The connection between two or more parts of the skeleton is called a joint. Joints enable the body to be flexible and to rotate.

For movement to occur, one or two main muscles contract, while at the same time, many other supporting muscles also contract or relax to some degree. As muscles contract and relax, joints are able to bend, enabling the body to move. If any bone, muscle or joint groups are not healthy, movement may be difficult and you could be at risk of breaking a bone by falling.

BONE BUILD-UP

Most of the skeleton in an unborn child is made up of cartilage – a dense connective tissue that is progressively replaced by calcified true bone. Throughout childhood, particularly during the rapid growth of adolescence, bone is formed at a greater rate than it is resorbed or lost.

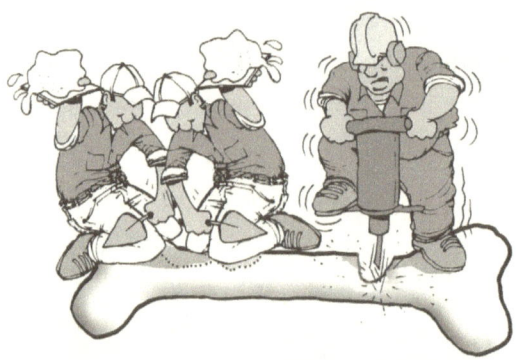

Throughout childhood, bone is formed at a greater rate than it is resorbed.

Bone strength occurs through a process known as remodeling. Remodeling helps to develop and maintain bone by taking away old bone and forming new bone. During this process, small holes are created by osteoclast (removal) cells. These holes are then filled in with new bone by osteoblasts (building) cells. At any one time, less than 1% of the bone is involved. This cycle of resorption or removal and formation of bone determines bone strength (density and quality).

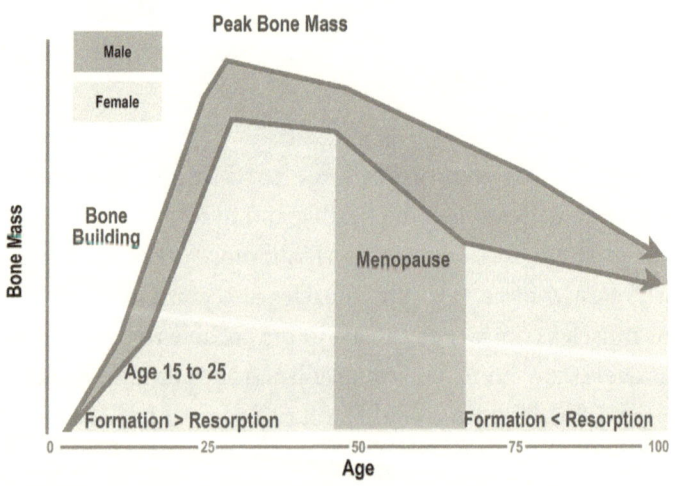

As a bone grows, it generally becomes more dense and stronger. Exercise and a diet rich in calcium and vitamin D help ensure you will have strong bones well into the future. Bone growth and development continues to about age 16-20 for females and about 20-25 for males, at which time peak bone mass is reached. Bone then stays relatively stable until the mid-thirties for both women and men.

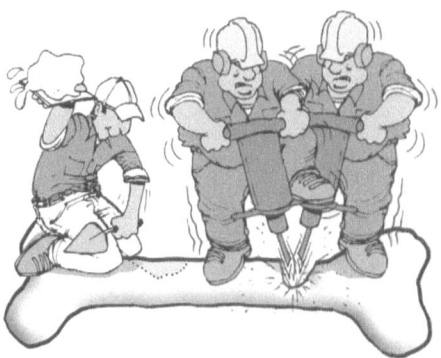

By our mid-thirties, the balance has shifted and more bone is resorbed than is formed

From about the mid-thirties, the balance naturally starts to shift. A little more bone (about 1%) is resorbed (removed) than is formed and bones may start to weaken. For women in menopause, bone loss is significantly higher due to the loss of estrogen. For five or six years around menopause, a woman can lose 1.5-3% of her bone density each year, increasing her risk of osteoporosis. As previously noted, when you have osteoporosis, your bones become weak, and weak bones increase the risk of fracture. Fractures often hurt and can leave people disabled. For the elderly, hip and spinal fractures can even lead to death.

HOW THE BODY MAINTAINS BONE

So how do our bodies maintain strong bones after we've reached peak bone mass? One way is through the food we eat. As digested foods are broken down, nutrients, such as calcium, phosphorus and some vitamin D, are absorbed into the bloodstream, mainly from the small intestine. As the bloodstream carries absorbed nutrients through the body, tissues take the nutrients they need. Generally, the body will not absorb more of a specific nutrient than it needs. If nutrients are not used immediately, they will be stored for use later or excreted by the body.

Detecting the amount of nutrients available is the role of certain hormone producing glands. Hormones involved in regulating blood calcium are:

- *parathyroid secreted by the parathyroid glands*
- *calcitonin from the thyroid gland*
- *calcitriol produced from vitamin D converted in the liver and in the kidney*

Other hormones that affect bone are:

- *thyroxine from the thyroid gland*
- *insulin from the pancreas*
- *growth hormone from the anterior pituitary gland*
- *cortisol from the adrenal glands*
- *estrogen and progesterone from the ovaries in women and fat tissue*
- *testosterone from the testes in men*

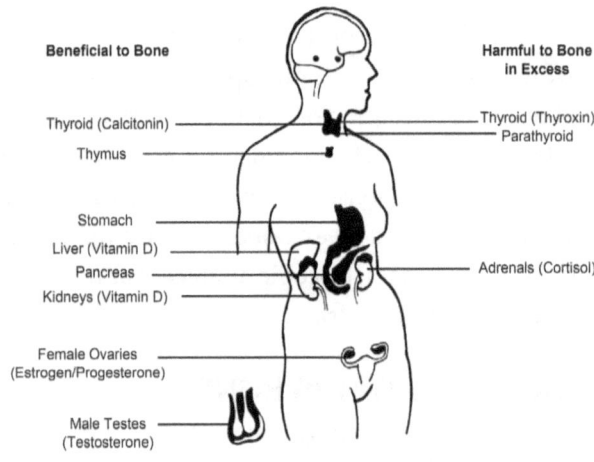

Glands and Hormones

Any condition that affects the absorption of nutrients or hormone-producing glands may affect the bones. Changes in the normal levels of hormones may cause a greater imbalance in bone formation and resorption, which can cause more bone to be removed than formed and thus weaken the bones. If you have any problems with your glandular (endocrine) system, discuss your bone health with your healthcare professional or a specialist in bone disease. If the problem is hormone related, your health-care professional may refer you to an endocrinologist.

The Impact of Genetics and Lifestyle on Your Bones

Genetics and lifestyle have significant influences on our bone health. Research suggests that genetic markers may identify some individuals who are at risk of developing osteoporosis. Testing people when they are younger and identifying individuals who are at high risk of osteoporosis may necessitate lifestyle changes, including taking medications to decrease the risk of fracture. Proper genetic testing is becoming less expensive, but remains somewhat inconclusive as to what actions will give the best outcome.

Stressors

As discussed earlier, there is a balance shift to more bone being removed than formed as we age. Bones then come under stress and can be at risk of fracture. The degree of risk depends on a person's original level of peak bone mass, the current strength of the bone and the amount of stress placed on it. Bone is influenced by four major stressors:

- *Mechanical stress, such as weight-bearing exercise, can enhance bone strength. Conversely, lack of resistance (e.g., being immobile) can result in bone loss.*
- *Hormonal stress caused by the loss of estrogen, testosterone or an imbalance of other hormones.*
- *Nutritional stress resulting from a diet deficient in adequate calcium, vitamin D and protein as well as some diseases of the gut.*
- *Aging that results naturally in more bone being removed than formed, leading to a decline in bone strength (density and quality).*

When bones cannot adapt to these stresses, they can become fragile and at increased risk of fracture.

THIN BONES AND FRACTURES

The human body has two types of bones: cortical and trabecular. Cortical bone, which is compact and dense, forms the outer shell of all bones. Trabecular bone, which is a less dense and spongier, is surrounded by harder cortical bone. The spine is largely composed of trabecular bone. Consequently, the spine is often the first area to show signs of bone loss and osteoporosis and is most vulnerable to fractures. The wrists, shoulders and hips are also vulnerable to fractures.

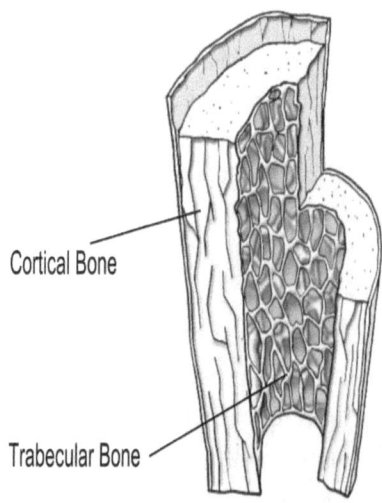

Cortical Bone

Trabecular Bone

Bone loss in the spine can cause the vertebrae to become weak and porous. Vertebrae can become so thin that they eventually collapse due to minor trauma, perhaps during a simple, everyday movement like lifting a bag of groceries. Amazingly, many people with collapsed vertebrae do not feel pain.

Collapsed vertebrae will also result in height loss and possibly an outward curve of the upper spine, known as kyphosis or dowager's hump, and an inward curve in the lower spine (lordosis) or a flat low back. You may also notice that your tummy sticks out a bit more. All of these are signs of fracture and osteoporosis.

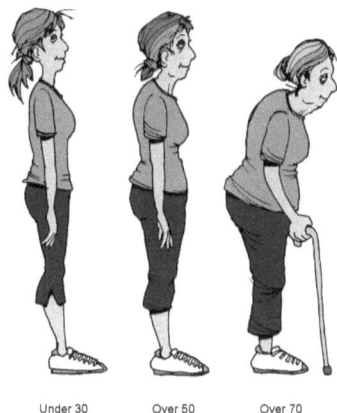

Collapsed Vertebrae Leading to a Curved Spine (Kyphosis)

Identifying Spinal Fractures

On the plus side, a spinal fracture or collapse can be identified on a chest X-ray or other radiograph, such as a spine X-ray (thoracic and lumbar). A patient can request that the bone health of the spine be checked when an X-ray is ordered. If a spinal fracture or collapse is evident, it should then be properly assessed for osteoporosis and treated to prevent future fractures. Surprisingly, a study of women over 60 who had a spine X-ray for a reason other than a suspected fracture (e.g., a chest X-ray for pneumonia) found that although almost half the women had spinal fractures, only 19% were identified and treated. When having a chest X-ray for any reason, ask your health-care professional to make a request to "rule out spinal fracture" on the X-ray.

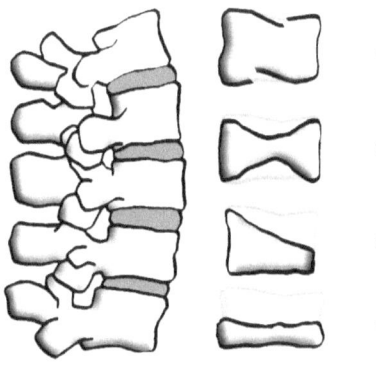

1.   End Plate Fracture

2.   Early Collapse (Concave)

3.   Wedged

4.   Crushed

Normal Vertebrae   Fractured Vertebrae

Keep Track of Your Height

Since height loss may be an indicator of osteoporosis and fractures in the spine, talk with your healthcare professional about a spinal fracture if you have had a height loss of:

- *2.5 inches (approximately 6 cm) since your tallest known height*
- *more than 1 inch (approximately 2.5 cm) in the last three years*

Although height loss is a simple and valuable way to detect vertebral fractures, it does not pick up all fractures or specify the type, such as a wedged or collapsed fracture. Height must be measured reliably and consistently to be of use in monitoring changes over time.

Hip Fractures

The most physically significant area for a fracture is the hip. Comprising 50% each of trabecular and cortical bone, the hip can fracture as result of a fall, although in some cases there is no apparent cause.

Hip fractures are associated with subsequent illnesses and mortality. More than one-quarter of women and more than one-third of men who suffer a hip fracture will die within one year, significantly higher than the death rate for a person without a fracture.

Wrist Fractures

Wrist fractures are more common at an earlier age and stage of osteoporosis. Wrist bones are made up mostly of trabecular bone (95%) and therefore are not as strong as other bones in the body. Wrist fractures occur frequently when the arm is extended to break a fall. Although not usually disabling, such a fracture can serve as a warning that extensive bone loss is occurring and there is increased risk of another fracture in the future. A healthcare professional might take this opportunity to further investigate your bone health.

Everyone's goal should be to prevent bone loss and osteoporosis before fractures occur rather than to treat them once they have occurred. Fortunately, there are steps you can take to slow bone loss before osteoporosis develops. We will look at these later in this book.

CAUSES OF BONE LOSS AND OSTEOPOROSIS

Of the many risk factors leading to bone loss and osteoporosis, most are generally categorized as either primary or secondary osteoporosis.

Primary Osteoporosis

Primary osteoporosis is when there is no obvious cause of bone loss other than changes due to genetics, age and/or post-menopause.

Post-menopausal Osteoporosis in Women

Bone loss is believed to be a result of a decrease in estrogen associated with menopause. Rapid bone loss of 1.5-3% a year occurs for five or six years around menopause before gradually slowing to 1% loss per year.

Age-related Osteoporosis in Men and Women

Bone loss naturally starts at a rate of 0.5-1% a year after a male or female reaches their mid-thirties; in other words, after their bones have reached their peak bone mass and stabilized.

Secondary Osteoporosis

Secondary osteoporosis is when immobility, disease or medications are identified as the cause of the bone loss or a fracture.

Immobility

Immobility can cause bone loss because there is no weight-bearing activity to stimulate bone formation. For example, astronauts are found to have bone loss while living in space. Due to the absence of gravity in space, without special equipment they are unable to bear weight and apply any stress directly to their bones. Back here on earth, a person might be immobile due to general inactivity or due to conditions such as rheumatoid arthritis, severe osteoarthritis, stroke, multiple sclerosis or spinal cord injury.

Disease

Disease can lead to an imbalance in bone resorption and bone formation and result in subsequent bone loss. Some of the more common diseases include:

- *celiac disease*
- *diabetes mellitus*
- *malabsorption of nutrients*
- *Crohn's disease*
- *Cushing's disease*
- *hypogonadism*
- *hyperthyroidism*
- *rheumatoid arthritis*
- *liver disease*
- *alcoholism*

If you have any of these conditions, talk with your healthcare professional about getting tested for bone loss. In all cases, measures to protect against bone loss should be started. Keep a close check on your height. Maintain a balanced lifestyle and a diet with adequate calcium, vitamin D (sunshine and supplements). And equally important, do regular strength, weight-bearing and balance exercises.

Medications

Due to their effect on bone remodeling, certain prescribed medications taken in low dosages over long periods of time can lead to bone loss. Examples include:

- *glucocorticoids (e.g., prednisone)*
- *thyroid hormones (in excessive doses)*
- *gonadotropin-releasing hormones (used to treat endometriosis in women and prostate cancer in men)*
- *anti-androgen therapy (used to treat benign prostate enlargement, some acne, male pattern baldness and excessive hairiness)*
- *aromatase inhibitors (used to treat breast cancer and ovarian cancer)*
- *proton pump inhibitors (e.g., Losec, Nexium)*
- *some seizure or anticonvulsant medications such as phenytoin (Dilantin), which can also increase risk of falling*

Glucocorticoid medications are the most serious cause of drug-induced osteoporosis and subsequent fracture risk. The most common glucocorticoid is prednisone, which is used to treat diseases associated with excessive inflammation.

Research suggests that glucocorticoid-induced osteoporosis can be prevented. Since bone loss is most rapid in the first six months of glucocorticoid use, preventive measures should begin immediately if therapy is expected to go beyond three months.

Consult your healthcare professional about any medications you are taking and their impact on possible bone loss, osteoporosis and fracture.

Betty's Story: Secondary Osteoporosis

Betty, a 55-year-old school teacher, has had rheumatoid arthritis for seven years. The disease is moderately active and she had been on low-dose prednisone for many years to control her symptoms. Since her doctor recently put her on a biologic medication, which she regularly self-injects, Betty has experienced dramatic improvement and has stopped taking the prednisone.

Rheumatoid arthritis is commonly associated with bone loss because of active inflammation, decreased physical activity and side-effects from medications such as prednisone. As Betty's rheumatoid arthritis has been active for seven years and she had been taking prednisone for a few years, she may be at high risk of future osteoporotic fractures.

Read about Betty's experience with secondary osteoporosis in Chapter 10.

Chapter 1 Key Points

- **Bone is a living tissue that is completely removed and replaced (known as remodeling) over a seven-year cycle.**
- **Peak bone mass is reached by age 16-20 for women and 20-25 for men.**
- **After reaching peak bone mass, bone stays stable until we reach our mid-thirties at which time we start to lose bone.**
- **Building a high peak bone mass is critically important to bone health.**
- **Certain nutrients and hormones help maintain our bones.**
- **Lifestyle and genetics influence our bone health.**

- The balance of bone building and bone removal (resorption) is affected by age.
- Some diseases and some medications adversely affect bone health. Steps should be taken to prevent or slow down bone loss if it is due to disease or medication.
- Discuss your bone health and height with your healthcare professional at each annual physical exam.

CHAPTER 2

Menopause and Bone Loss

Menopause occurs when a woman's ovaries no longer produce estrogen and progesterone. The loss of estrogen can increase the rate of bone loss and therefore increase a woman's risk of fracture.

CALLING ALL WOMEN

Menopause, which is 12 consecutive months without menstruation, can begin when a woman reaches her mid-forties. In North America, the average age is 51.

Menopause is not the only reason why the menstrual cycle may stop. Extreme athletics, pregnancy, radiation or surgical removal of ovaries can also lead to a change in your menstrual cycle. If your menstrual cycle stops, do not assume that you are in beginning stages of menopause. As with any changes in your menstrual cycle, it is important to consult with your healthcare professional to identify or confirm why these changes are happening in your body.

COMMON SIGNS AND SYMPTOMS OF MENOPAUSE

- *irregular periods that eventually result in no menstruation within 9-12 months*
- *hot flushes, night sweats, frequent urination and/or insomnia*
- *unusual irritability, headaches or depression*
- *vaginal dryness or changes in sexual desire*

Managing menopausal symptoms can be confusing as well as controversial. Issues arise in regards to using pharmaceutical medicines or compounded preparations or herbal remedies or doing nothing.

Hormone therapy often provides some symptom relief as well as protection against bone loss and fracture. This protection stops when the hormone therapy stops. Adequate calcium and vitamin D supplementation along with regular strength and weight-bearing exercises are also important in maintaining bone health.

WHY BONE LOSS?

As we age, we lose bone. However, women lose bone at a faster rate than men due to menopause. A woman can naturally lose as much as 18% of her bone mass during menopause. By the time a woman is 80, she may have lost up to 45% of her bone. Whereas a man of the same age might have lost 25% of his bone.

Bone loss as a result of menopause is related to loss of estrogen and progesterone. Estrogen is the main sex hormone in women and helps block the bone-dissolving action of the parathyroid hormone. One of the functions of progesterone is to balance the effects of estrogen. With the onset of menopause, the ovaries no longer produce these hormones and the body is less likely to maintain the equilibrium between bone formation and resorption. As women lose estrogen, the increased rate of bone loss should be a concern. As noted in Chapter 1, menopause can account for a woman losing 1.5-3% of her bone per year and, depending on her original peak bone mass, increase her risk of developing osteoporosis.

Women close to the age of menopause may want to discuss possible treatments with their healthcare professional. The most common treatment is hormone therapy, but it is not without its controversies. The Women's Health Initiative, a 15-year study of 161,808 women aged 50-79 study, found a number of benefits and risks associated with therapies involving estrogen and progesterone or estrogen alone compared with placebo.

While there is evidence that the amount of bone may increase during the first few years of therapy, bone protection is considered an additional benefit, not usually the main reason for hormones therapy.

Be your own best advocate. Learn all you can from trustworthy sources and then talk with your healthcare professional about your personal beliefs about menopause, medical history and bone health status.

Chapter 2 Key Points

- Estrogen plays a significant role in preventing bone loss.

- Women can take steps to slow bone loss through adequate calcium, vitamin D and weight-bearing exercises.

- Discuss your bone health options with your healthcare professional before you start to experience symptoms of menopause.

- Hormone therapy provides relief for some menopausal symptoms.

- Women may experience rapid bone loss during the first six years of menopause.

- Bone protection is considered an additional benefit and not usually the main reason for hormone therapy.

Testosterone, Age-related Hypogonadism and Bone Loss

Hypogonadism (low testosterone) is a risk factor for osteoporosis. Diagnosing hypogonadism can be challenging.

Robert's Story: Men and Osteoporosis

Robert, 55, broke his right wrist when he fell rushing across a parking lot. Robert has always had a poor diet. He smokes a pack of cigarettes a day despite having asthma. Treatment for his asthma has included inhaled steroid puffers and frequent short courses of prednisone during flares. His doctor recognizes risk factors for future fractures and osteoporosis and advises Robert to have a bone mineral density test and complete a fracture risk assessment.

CALLING ALL MEN

Low testosterone is one of several risk factors for osteoporosis and fracture in men. It is estimated that:

- *10% of men over 50 experience symptoms of low testosterone*
- *1 in 5 men over 50 suffer from low bone density or osteoporosis*
- *by age 50, a man has a 13% chance of a fracture due to weak bones*
- *by 60, that fracture risk increases to 25%*
- *25% of all hip fractures occur among elderly males*

Signs and symptoms of low testosterone are often vague and vary significantly from one man to another. Some men describe the feeling by stating: "I used to be a jock and now I am a couch potato." Symptoms can be broadly grouped as:

- *low sex drive*
- *fewer or weaker erections*
- *emotional, psychological and behaviour changes*

- *muscle aches and reduced muscle strength*
- *increased upper and central body fat*
- *decline in general well-being and energy level*
- *mental fatigue and reduced ability to concentrate*

Unlike the rapid decline in estrogen experienced by females during menopause, the loss of testosterone among aging men is gradual (about 1% loss/year after the age of 30). Blood tests for free and total testosterone, and sex hormone-binding globulin (SHBG) can measure the level of a man's testosterone.

A significant decline in testosterone is neither universal nor experienced by all aging males. Hypogonadism is a condition in which the body does not produce enough sex hormones. Generally, age-related hypogonadism in men is the result of low testosterone and can reach a point where the level of testosterone is so low that it causes medical symptoms that require correcting. Hypogonadism may be the result of certain prostate cancer therapies, the removal of testicles, or the result of the testicles being normal but functioning improperly.

Testosterone replacement therapy should be considered on an individual basis. If you have been diagnosed with moderate to severe bone loss or have a fragility fracture, then there are more appropriate therapies to treat your bone loss. Talk to your healthcare professional.

Testosterone replacement therapy should not be confused with treatments used for erectile dysfunction – for example taking sildenafil (Viagra), tadalafil (Cialis) or vardenafil (Levitra). These treatments help to produce erections in men with erectile dysfunction regardless of testosterone level, and do not have any effect on bone loss.

Read about Robert's experience with osteoporosis in Chapter 10.

Chapter 3 Key Points

- Osteoporosis in older men is common.

- Men can take steps to slow bone loss through adequate calcium, vitamin D and weight-bearing exercises.

- Men lose about 1% testosterone/year after the age of 30 and may become noticeable as men get older. Some may have significant signs and symptoms of low testosterone such as persistent lack of energy, decreased interest in sex, weak erections, sadness or grumpiness.

- Hypogonadism (low testosterone) is one of several important risk factors for bone loss in men.

- Twenty-five percent of hip fractures occur among elderly males.

- Testosterone replacement therapy may, on an individual basis, be considered for men with hypogonadism.

CHAPTER 4

Preventing Falls and Fractures

When an adult breaks a bone – think osteoporosis!

FALLS

- *The first objective in preventing fractures due to falls is to prevent a fall from occurring. This might sound obvious, but falls often happen when they could have been avoided by safeguarding the environment around you and doing exercises targeted at improving balance and strength.*

- *The second objective is to prevent broken bones from occurring if you fall. By having the best bone density, structure and quality of bone, you will reduce your risk of fracture from a fall.*

More than one-third of adults over the age of 65 fall each year. Falls are the most common cause of injury among the elderly. One third of people who fall suffer moderate to severe injuries such as bruising, head trauma, broken wrists or hip fractures. Falls account for 40% of elderly admissions to nursing homes and long-term care facilities. Elderly people who experience a fall often fear they might fall again. This fear may lead to anxiety causing the person to limit their movements and become overcautious and tense, which in turn can increase the risk of falling again.

RISK FACTORS FOR FALLS AND FRACTURES

Low bone density is one risk factor for osteoporosis-related broken bones. Other factors you should be aware of include:

- *age, the risk of fracture increases with age, especially at 65 years and older*
- *decreased sight, hearing, balance or muscle strength*
- *prior fragility (low trauma, low impact) fracture*
- *poor health status – frail*
- *balance – unstable on your feet*

- *experiencing two or more falls in the last year*
- *experienced a fracture after age 40*
- *family history of osteoporotic fracture (e.g., parental hip fracture; spine fracture, stooped posture}*
- *long-term use of glucocorticoid (more than three months continuously) therapy such as prednisone that can affect your muscles and bones so they become weak*
- *medications that affect your mobility and balance, such as sedatives*
- *dizziness or bouts of low blood pressure, especially blood pressure medications at too high of a dose*
- *environmental hazards, such as uneven pavement on sidewalks, loose area rugs, poor lighting*

Keeping muscles strong and staying agile and supple will help to prevent falls and fractures from occurring. Because an older person has lower bone density, resulting in weaker bones, the amount of stress required to cause a break may be much less than for a younger person. A small fall or even an unexpected twist can result in a fracture, which is why balance and balance exercises are very important as we age.

If you fall, your risk of breaking a bone may depend on one or more of the following:

- *your height*
- *the distance of your fall*
- *any protective response, such as putting your hand out to break a fall*
- *the type of surface on which you fall*
- *the angle in which you fall; falling sideways or straight down is riskier than falling backwards*
- *bone geometry or shape and density of your bone*
- *whether or not you were wearing a good hip protector that fits properly*

FRACTURE PREVENTION

A broken bone is often the first sign that an older person has osteoporosis. Unfortunately, by the time the fracture occurs, the osteoporosis is well advanced and the individual runs a 20% chance of another fracture within the next 12 months.

Time after time, osteoporosis, the underlying cause of many fractures, goes undetected. There is a lack of attention and treatment given to people who have had an osteoporosis-related fracture. They are often sent home without any treatment or measures in place to prevent another fracture from occurring, even though these people have been shown to be at the highest risk to suffer another fracture.

Fracture Liaison Service

Fortunately, a growing number of hospitals and outpatient clinics are establishing a fracture liaison service. This ensures that patients who present at a hospital or clinic with a fracture receive secondary or future fracture risk assessments and treatment as appropriate.

The main objectives of a fracture liaison service include:

- *Identification. A primary care provider who has taken responsibility for the patient's care is alerted that the fracture has occurred and further assessment is needed.*
- *Investigation. The care provider investigates the fragility fracture, requesting, if necessary, laboratory tests and risk assessments making the diagnosis of osteoporosis.*
- *Initiation. Osteoporosis treatment is provided as appropriate keeping in mind to include lifestyle measures as well as discuss appropriate drug therapies.*

MOBILITY AIDS

If you are unsteady on your feet and have a fear of falling, you have some choices. You can remain active by using a good supportive walking shoe or hiking boot along with a mobility aid, such as a cane or walker, to provide safer, more secure movement, or you can accept a less physically active life with fewer social interactions, increased health risks and a reduced quality of life. If you are self-conscious, remember a mobility aid can help you maintain or improve your quality of life.

Chapter 4 Key Points

- If you break a bone after age 40, think osteoporosis and follow up with your healthcare professional.

- Fewer than 20% of women and 10% of men are appropriately tested after an osteoporotic-related fracture.

- If you break a bone, see if there is a fracture liaison service that you should be enrolled with.

- Be aware of the effects that age, disease, medications, lifestyle and environment may have on your risk of falling.

- Keeping your muscles strong and staying agile and supple will help prevent falls and fractures.

- Be aware of your height and any height loss as loss may signal a spine fracture.

- Take steps to prevent another fall and fracture. Do weight-bearing and balance exercises and use osteoporosis medication and mobility aids such as canes or walkers as necessary.

CHAPTER 5

Preventing Osteoporosis

While there is no cure for osteoporosis, there are non-pharmacological ways to slow down bone loss and the onset of osteoporosis through diet and exercise.

Earlier, we pointed out that your family health history may be an indicator that you might be at risk of osteoporosis. We also noted that lifestyle has a significant impact on bone development. In this chapter, we identify foods that are high in calcium or that affect calcium absorption. We offer suggestions on how to adjust your diet to improve calcium absorption and we discuss the value of vitamin D and other vitamins and minerals. If you are unable to get enough vitamin D or dietary calcium (e.g., you are on a vegan diet or have celiac disease), you will learn how supplements can help you meet your daily requirements.

DIET AND BONE HEALTH

A well-balanced diet should provide your body with the necessary fats, carbohydrates, proteins, water, mineral salts and vitamins. National daily food guides are designed to help ensure that all nutrients are obtained in a proper balance to meet our basic nutritional needs. Carbohydrates, fats and proteins provide the body with the calories that produce the body's energy and building blocks. Electrolytes, water, vitamins and minerals are important for cellular build-up and break-down that occurs in the body. Not all foods are equal in the nutrition they offer, so some foods receive more attention in food guides. Food guides, such as the United States' *MyPlate Food Guidance System* and *Canada's Food Guide* are available online, through your library, from healthcare professionals, registered dietitians and health clinics.

Your body has several built-in regulating mechanisms or checks and balances. A change in one thing will likely affect something else. The change may be for better or worse, but the result of the change may take months or years to show up. Consider how slowly the body builds bone. For women, bone keeps building until the late teens and for men until the mid-twenties. If we maintained an optimal well-balanced healthy diet during our younger years and got plenty of exercise, the risk of developing osteoporosis later in life would be reduced.

Minerals (e.g., calcium, phosphorus, magnesium) and vitamins (e.g., vitamins D, A, K) are important in bone health. With the exception of vitamin D, minerals and vitamins are more than adequately covered in a varied, well-balanced, healthy diet, provided your body absorbs the nutrients properly.

CALCIUM

The body needs calcium for:

- *strong teeth and bones*
- *nerve and muscle function*
- *maintaining cell permeability (the passage of fluids through the cell walls)*
- *regulating blood pressure and maintaining normal heart rate and rhythm*
- *blood clotting*

If our daily diet does not include enough calcium, or if calcium is not absorbed properly in our bodies, our blood calcium levels decrease. The parathyroid gland, which is responsible for controlling the calcium in our blood and bones, will then send out more parathyroid hormone, causing the bones to release more calcium into the bloodstream. If this continues over a long period of time, bones become brittle and at greater risk of fracturing. This risk of fracture is from low bone density and is discussed in Chapter 7.

Calcium has an important role in the prevention and treatment of osteoporosis. The daily recommended amount of calcium in an average person's diet is 1,000-2,000 mg, depending on age, gender and medical history. About 75% of the calcium in an average diet comes from dairy products. Eating calcium-rich foods is the best way to ensure that calcium is always available when your body needs it. Many people don't consume enough dairy products and find it difficult to maintain a diet that meets the recommended daily calcium intake.

Although dairy products are the richest sources of calcium, fortified rice or soy beverages contain the equivalent amount of calcium as found in milk – 8 oz/250 ml equals about 320 mg of calcium. For people who have trouble tolerating milk, adding the enzyme lactase to milk helps break down the milk sugar and may improve the ability to digest milk. If you have an allergy to dairy products or choose to avoid them, discuss your diet and need for calcium supplements with your healthcare professional. Calcium supplements and non-dairy foods containing calcium are discussed later in this chapter.

Certain foods, diseases and medications can affect the amount of calcium the stomach and intestines are able to draw into the bloodstream from the food you eat. The following can result in the depletion of some nutrients in your body. If any of these apply to you, consider adjusting your diet or taking supplements:

- *Not eating a well-balanced diet. As we age, we may eat too little and have a poor diet, such as just taking tea and toast. Some younger people may be constantly dieting or be anorexic or bulimic.*
- *Food allergies that prevent you from getting the necessary nutrients.*
- *Glands that over-produce or under-produce hormones that impact calcium levels.*
- *Digestive problems {e.g., resulting from celiac disease, Crohn's disease, diarrhea, bariatric surgery).*
- *Medications that impact the digestive system, which can cause malabsorption of nutrients.*

If you have a history of kidney stones, precautions should be considered. A good work-up or medical assessment from your healthcare professional or specialist should help to rule out any underlying causes or factors that impact how much calcium you should take.

Calcium Intake

The following checklist will give you an approximate calculation of your dietary calcium intake. If you are low or borderline, you may want to do a more detailed calculation with your healthcare professional, nurse practitioner or registered dietitian. Websites of national osteoporosis organizations and most dairy foundations also offer methods to calculate calcium.

Libraries and your healthcare professional also have charts to calculate your calcium intake.

QUICK CALCIUM INTAKE CHECKLIST

Here is a simple way to calculate your calcium intake:

- *List all the foods you eat in a day. For a more accurate reflection, list the foods you eat over three days and include a weekend when your diet may be different from your usual weekdays.*
- *List the foods in easily measurable amounts, such as cups, ounces or milligrams.*
- *Use the food charts on the following pages (or any other food chart) and list the milligrams (mg) of calcium in each food. Some foods do not contain significant amounts of calcium and are not listed here. Consider the amount of calcium that these foods contribute as a bonus to your daily calcium intake.*
- *Add up the amounts. Be sure to check serving sizes and milligrams, then adjust as necessary. Compare your amounts with the recommendations for your age group.*

When counting your calcium intake, consider both dietary intake and supplements. Do not forget to include multivitamins. The National Osteoporosis Foundation and Osteoporosis Canada recommend:

Age	Calcium mg/day
4-8	800 mg
9-19	1,300 mg
20-50	1,000 mg
50+	1,200 mg*

*Many adults only consume 300-700 mg/day of calcium. A well-balanced non-milk diet often contains 300 mg of calcium. Some experts recommend up to 1,500 mg/day of calcium

Many suggest the safe upper limit for a total calcium intake should not exceed 1,500-1,800 mg/day unless you have malabsorption issues or unless your healthcare professional or dietitian recommends otherwise. Research is also showing that individuals over the age of 50 who have sufficient vitamin D intake (which helps with calcium absorption) require a total calcium intake of 800-1,200 mg/day. If your primary source of calcium is from foods other than milk products, you may need to consume a large quantity of these foods in order to meet the recommended daily requirement of calcium.

The calcium you get from the food you eat is best. However, if food does not provide you with an adequate amount of calcium, you may need a calcium supplement. But remember, more calcium is not always better. While calcium is important, too much calcium may be harmful.

The following charts cluster foods into categories based on their calcium content. It is important to know the general amount of calcium rather than the specific amount; hence the figures are in round numbers rather than specific amounts. An 8 oz/250 ml glass of milk contains about 320 mg of calcium and 100 IU of vitamin D. Similarly, an 8 oz/250 ml glass of fortified orange juice and soy beverage also contains about 320 mg of calcium. Therefore, drinking two glasses of milk a day is a good start towards meeting your daily calcium requirements. If vegetables are your main source of calcium, you will need to eat a lot more of the vegetables listed in these charts to get the recommended daily requirement of calcium.

300-500 MG CALCIUM/SERVING

Food	Estimated Serving
Beans: Black	1 cup/250 ml
Bok Choy: Cooked	1 cup/250 ml
Cheese: Brick, Caraway, Colby, Edam	1.5 oz/45 g
Cheese: Ricotta (skimmed milk)	1 cup/250 ml
Cheese: Farmers, Swiss	1.5 oz/45 g
Macaroni and Cheese	1 cup/250 ml
Beverages: Fortified Rice, Soy, Almond,	1 cup/250 ml
Milk: Evaporated, Undiluted (2%, skim, whole)	1 cup/250 ml
Milk: Powdered Skim	4 tbsp/60 ml
Milk: Buttermilk, Chocolate	1 cup/250 ml
Orange Juice (Fortified)	1 cup/250 ml
Sardines with Bones	3 oz/90 g
Tofu: in Calcium Sulfate	1 cup/250ml
Yogurt: Plain, Skim	6oz/180ml

200-300 MG CALCIUM/SERVING

Food	Estimated Serving
Cheese: Blue, Feta, Mozzarella	1.5 oz/45 g
Cheese: Parmesan	3 tbsp/100 g
Cheese: Processed	1.5 oz/45 g
Ice Cream Sundae	1 cup/250 ml
Milk: Powdered, Whole	4 tbsp/ 60ml
Salmon: Canned, Drained, with bones	0.5 cup/125 ml

100-200 MG CALCIUM/SERVING

Food	Estimated Serving
Almonds	1.5 oz/45 g
Baked Beans with Tomato Sauce	1 cup/250 ml
Brazil Nuts	0.5 cup/125 ml
Broccoli Cooked	1 cup/250 ml
Cheese: Cottage 4%, skim	1 cup/250 ml
Chile Con Carne and Beans	1 cup/250 ml
Cream of Wheat Cooked	1 cup/250 ml
Custard Baked	0.5 cup/125 ml
Custard Pie	1 wedge
English Muffin with Egg, Cheese and Bacon	1
Figs: Dried, 5 Medium	3 oz/90 g
Ice Cream	0.75 cup/185 ml
Kale	0.5 cup/125 ml
Lobster	3 oz/90 g
Molasses: Blackstrap/Cooking	1 tbsp/15 ml
Pizza with Cheese	1 piece
Pudding: Instant, Rice, Tapioca	0.5 cup/125 ml
Sesame Seeds	0.5 cup/125 ml
Shrimp	28 med. size
Soup: Cream of Chicken, Mushroom, Tomato	1 cup/250 ml
Soy Beans	1 cup/250 ml
Spaghetti and Meat Sauce	1 cup/250 ml
White Beans	1 cup/250 ml

UNDERSTANDING FOOD LABELS

When reading a label, look for the calcium content. The percentage (%) of daily value (DV) or percentage of recommended daily intake (RDI) noted on a label is generally based on approximately 1,000 mg of calcium/day. So, a label stating "calcium 10%" would mean that one serving contains 100 mg of calcium. Be sure to read the label and note the amount of a "serving size."

Nutrition Facts

Serving Size 172g

Amount Per Serving	
Calories 200	Calories from Fat 8

	% Daily Value*
Total Fat 1g	1%
Saturated Fat 0g	1%
Trans Fat	
Cholesterol 0mg	0%
Sodium 6mg	0%
Total Carbohydrate 36g	12%
Dietary Fiber 11g	45%
Sugars 6g	
Protein 13g	

Vitamin A	1%	Vitamin C	1%
Calcium	4%	Iron	24%

*Percent Daily Values are based on a 2,000 calorie diet. Your daily values may be higher or lower depending on your calorie needs.

FOODS THAT ROB BONES OF CALCIUM

Some foods can rob your bones of calcium. Calcium robbers are foods that are high in oxalates and phytates – antinutrients that reduce the absorption of nutrients in digestive system. Regular servings of such foods are good for you and do not pose a threat. However, when taken in large quantities, these foods may interfere or block absorption of calcium. Do not stop eating these foods, but try to avoid eating them with foods you depend on for calcium. Alternatively, you can increase your calcium intake at the time you eat these foods.

Here are some tips to help manage these issues:

- *Eat a variety of vegetables to balance out the oxalates. Foods containing oxalates, such as rhubarb, spinach, beet greens and Swiss chard, carry valuable minerals and vitamins that your body needs.*

- *Foods containing phytates, such as pita bread, navy beans, kidney beans, peas, and wheat and bran cereals, have valuable nutrients. Increase your calcium intake in other ways when you eat these foods by adding, for example, a slice of cheese or a glass of milk.*

- *Eat small amounts of protein with every meal rather than one large serving a day. Too much protein may increase calcium loss through your kidneys. However, the body needs protein to function effectively.*

- *Drink another glass of milk a few hours after your meal to ensure you get the required calcium. Fiber should be a part of a well-balanced diet. However, the amount of calcium from a high-fiber meal may not provide the amount of calcium you need.*
- *Be aware of your salt intake. In addition to contributing to high blood pressure, salt added to your meals and the processed foods you eat may cause calcium loss through your kidneys.*
- *Caffeine contributes to the loss of calcium by excreting it through the urine. Replace coffee, cola drinks and some energy drinks with non-caffeine beverages, such as flavored milk or hot chocolate. Avoid drinking more than three cups of coffee per day. To increase calcium intake, add milk.*

INCREASE DIETARY CALCIUM

It is important to consider the foods that can block calcium absorption or rob you of calcium during digestion. Be aware of opportunities to increase calcium in your daily meal preparation. Here are some easy ways to increase the calcium content of your food:

Add:
- *dry-milk powder to fluid milk; one-third cup of powder per 1 cup milk will double the calcium content (1 teaspoon contains about 50 mg of calcium)*
- *cheese to casseroles, vegetable dishes, popcorn, toast, sandwiches*
- *cooked soybeans to soup, mayonnaise and seasoning to make a sandwich spread*

Substitute:
- *low-fat milk for water in most soups, drink mixes and baked products*
- *yogurt for sour cream*
- *yogurt and dry milk powder for mayonnaise*
- *desserts, such as rice puddings, tapioca, custards and bread puddings, for pastries, cakes and other foods high in fat*
- *skim ricotta cheese for cottage cheese*
- *soybeans for other kinds of beans in a recipe*

General:

- *Use tofu that has been prepared with calcium sulfate rather than calcium salt or magnesium (read the label).*
- *Drink milk shakes or hot milk flavored with cinnamon, cloves, almond extract or a small amount of decaffeinated coffee instead of soft drinks or regular coffee.*
- *Use roasted soybeans to enhance a snack recipe.*
- *Drink orange juice fortified with calcium and vitamin D.*

High Calcium Diets

People who have diets high in calcium, particularly diets that are high in dairy products, may encounter problems such as lactose intolerance, constipation and high fat intake.

LACTOSE INTOLERANCE

To be properly digested, milk sugar (lactose) in dairy products must be broken down by the enzyme lactase. Some people are not able to produce enough of this enzyme, which may result in bloating, abdominal cramping, diarrhea, nausea, vomiting and gas. These symptoms usually appear 30 minutes to two hours after ingesting lactose. This is not an allergy or immune response to milk, but if you are concerned, talk with your healthcare professional about the availability and cost of a breath hydrogen test for lactose intolerance.

Before you completely avoid milk products, you may wish to try some of the following tips.

Tips:

- *Consume only small amounts of milk products at any one time (2-4 oz/60-12 5ml).*
- *Consume milk products in combination with other ingredients or foods.*
- *Consume milk products, such as hard cheeses, that contain very little lactose.*
- *Drink milk that is heated.*
- *Use yogurt in food preparation. Yogurt contains high amounts of bacterial cultures that contain lactase.*

- *Add dry-milk powder to soups, casseroles, baking and so forth.*
- *Talk to a healthcare professional about the use of lactase enzymes (Lactaid) or other commercially available lactase enzymes. When added to milk, lactase enzymes break down the sugar and help in the digestion of milk.*

CONSTIPATION AND GAS

Having regular bowel movements means you move your bowels from 1-3 times/day or three times/week so long as that is your usual pattern. As we learn more about the importance of our gut, try to maintain regular bowel habits.

If constipation or gas is an issue for you, eating more foods high in fiber, such as raw fruit, vegetables and bran, may help counteract the constipation. However, consistently eating large servings of foods very high in fiber will tend to decrease the absorption of calcium. Since fiber in your diet is good, try to take small amounts more frequently during the day. Use a food guide to know your fiber requirements and to gradually increase your fiber intake as needed.

Tips:
- *Drink water (6-8 glasses per day).*
- *Use natural laxatives, such as prune juice, figs, chia seeds, flax seeds.*
- *Eat fruits and vegetables high in roughage, such as apples, celery, corn, dried beans and peas.*
- *Laxatives work in different ways, so talk with your pharmacist about safe, effective temporary use of over-the-counter laxatives.*

HIGH FAT INTAKE

Low-fat and high-fat foods are comparable in calcium content. If you want to decrease your fat intake, be selective about the foods you choose and look at the percentage of fat they contain. Low-fat milk products are often a good choice.

Tips:
- *Avoid fried foods and cream sauces.*

- *If cholesterol is not an issue, hard cheeses are higher in calcium and, therefore, a good choice. Choose foods that are low in fat, such as skim or 1% milk, low-fat yogurt or 1% cottage cheese over 4% cottage cheese.*
- *Eat a variety of fruits and vegetables. These are low in fat and are a good source of other necessary nutrients.*

Calcium Supplements

As we age, our dietary intake may change for any number of reasons. As previously noted, research shows that individuals 50 and older generally have a daily intake of only 300-700 mg of calcium from dietary sources, which is less than the recommended 1,200 mg/day from all sources.

Earlier we showed you a simple way to calculate how much calcium you get every day using the Quick Calcium Intake Checklist. Another method for finding out how much calcium you are getting from your diet is the Calcium Rule of 300, which is recommended by American Bone Health and other organizations.

Calcium Rule of 300

Number of daily 300 mg servings of dairy = _____

X 300 mg = _____

+   300

Calcium from diet = _____ mg

Food remains the best source of calcium and milk products are the easiest dietary source of calcium. If you have tried to improve your calcium intake and still do not reach the recommended daily amount, then you may want to consider taking oral calcium supplements. There are two main types of calcium supplements:

- *Calcium carbonate (most common) is 40% elemental calcium and must be taken with food.*
- *Calcium citrate is 21% elemental calcium and does not need to be taken with food.*

Elemental calcium is the actual amount of calcium in the supplement available for the body to absorb. Only about 500 mg of elemental calcium is absorbed at a time. Any supplement greater than 500 mg of elemental calcium will not be absorbed by the body. If you need more than 500 mg supplementation, take one dose in the morning and the remaining dosage in the afternoon.

When choosing a supplement, be sure the product is consistent and offers pure content, is easy to digest and tolerate, and is convenient to take and adequately absorbed. Read the label and note serving size for the amount of calcium supplementation you need to add to your dietary intake in order to meet your daily calcium requirement.

Some supplements offer a combination of vitamins and minerals, such as magnesium, phosphorus and vitamins D and K. Combination products rarely have the right amounts of all the vitamins and minerals that you, as an individual, need. Get advice about supplements from your pharmacist or healthcare professional.

VITAMIN D

Known as the sunshine vitamin, vitamin D is essential in calcium and phosphorus metabolism and is required for normal development of bones and teeth. It is an important part of bone health and in the prevention and treatment of osteoporosis.

Most experts recommend that adults under 50 need 600-1,000 international units (IU) of vitamin D supplementation per day and people over 50 need about 800-2,000 IU/day supplementation. More recent guidelines recommend supplementation of up to 2,000 IU/day. For people who do not have a vitamin D deficiency, doses above 2,000 IU/day have not been demonstrated to be better. Intakes of 4,000-6,000 IU/day may be safe, but there is no clear benefit in taking this higher dose. Furthermore, excessive amounts of vitamin D may cause a build up of calcium in your blood which can lead to kidney problems.

A blood test known as 25-OH vitamin D is the best way to know if you're getting enough vitamin D. Generally, 20-30 nanograms/milliliter (ng/ml) – or the metric equivalent of 50 nanomoles/liter (nmoles/l) – is considered an adequate blood level for vitamin D. Within this range, parathyroid hormone (PTH) is controlled to enable maximum calcium absorption and, thus, improve bone health and reduce fracture risk. Levels below 12 ng/l (30 nmol/l) indicate a significant vitamin D deficiency.

Vitamin D Intake

Vitamin D comes from three main sources:

- *skin's exposure to the sun*
- *dietary intake*
- *supplements*

Sunshine is considered the best, most efficient source of vitamin D. Vitamin D3 is naturally produced in your skin when it is exposed to sunlight. Most experts agree that depending on your location, season, time of day and angle of the sun, arms and legs exposed to sun with no sunscreen for 15-20 minutes a day will provide about 3,000 IU of vitamin D, more than the required daily dose of vitamin D for most people. However, be aware that excessive exposure to the sun may increase the risk of skin cancer and wrinkled or dry skin.

Few foods naturally contain or are fortified with vitamin D. Natural food sources of vitamin D include fatty fish, fish liver oils and egg yolks. Foods fortified with vitamin D include butter, cereal, cheese, margarine, milk, orange juice and yogurt.

VITAMIN D/ FOOD SERVING

Food	Serving	Vitamin D (est.)
Fresh wild salmon	3.5 oz/100 g	750 IU
Canned salmon	3.5 oz/100 g	450 IU
Canned mackerel or sardines	3.5 oz /100 g	360 IU
Fresh farmed salmon	3.5 oz/100 g	200 IU
Canned tuna in oil	3.5 oz/100 g	200 IU
Margarine	1 tbsp/15 ml	90 IU
Milk, fortified or enriched soy or rice beverage	1 cup/250 ml	90 IU
Egg yolk	1	20 IU

Vitamin D Supplements

Because adequate sun exposure is not always possible due to climate and geography, supplementation is one way to make sure you get enough vitamin D. Vitamin D supplements can be either vitamin D2 or D3, which are similar.

Vitamin D3 supplements are manufactured from animal sources while vitamin D2 comes from some plants and fortified foods. Vitamin D3 is thought to be more than three times as effective as the same amount of vitamin D2 in affecting blood levels and maintaining those levels longer.

While most multivitamins or calcium supplements contain some vitamin D, the amounts can vary and may not be adequate for reaching your daily requirement. As noted above, vitamin D levels can be checked by a blood test.

OTHER VITAMINS AND MINERALS

Vitamin A

Vitamin A is a fat-soluble vitamin essential for normal growth and development of eyes, teeth, bones and tissues that form the skin and line the body cavities. It also helps the body resist infection. Too much vitamin A, however, can actually cause bone loss. The daily requirement of vitamin A for men and post-menopausal women is about 2,500 IU or less. Menstruating women require a little more vitamin A, but still less than 5,000 IU/day.

There are two types of vitamin A: retinoids, from which retinol derives, comes from animal sources; and carotenoids, which includes beta-carotene, the precursor to vitamin A comes from plant foods. Research has found that high daily intake of supplemental retinol vitamin A (greater than 2,000 IU/day) affects bone remodeling and can be associated with an increased risk of hip fractures. However, beta-carotene vitamin A does not have the same associated risk of hip fractures or increased risk of osteoporosis.

Vitamin K

Vitamin K plays a role in bone metabolism and is a potential protector against osteoporosis. People who form blood clots too quickly or easily, and who may be taking a drug such as warfarin (Coumadin) should be routinely monitored by their healthcare professional. Warfarin can work to decrease the activity of vitamin K and lengthen the time it takes for a clot to form. However, this anticoagulant may also negatively affect bone health and steps should be taken to optimize your bones. If you are taking a blood thinner, know your vitamin K intake and keep it consistent from day to day. Work with your healthcare professional to best manage your treatment and protect your bone health.

As with most dietary vitamins, vitamin K is obtained through a varied and well-balanced diet. Vitamin K is found in beef liver, green tea, turnip greens, broccoli, kale, cabbage, asparagus and dark green and leafy vegetables. The average suggested daily requirement of vitamin K is about 90 micrograms (mcg) for women and 120 mcg for men. Just 0.5 cup/125ml of broccoli provides more than twice the daily requirement of vitamin K.

Sometimes you might see K1 and K2, which are the compounds that make up vitamin K. Some people use vitamin K2 to treat osteoporosis. However, to date there is no scientific evidence to support this, so vitamin K is not currently recommended as a treatment.

Phosphorus

Phosphorus is a mineral that combines with calcium to form the hard structure of your bones and teeth. It requires vitamin D for its absorption and metabolism. Normally excreted by the kidneys and intestines, an excessive amount of phosphorus in the body is rare, but too much phosphorous interferes with calcium uptake. A healthy diet has enough phosphorus-containing foods to meet the roughly 800 mg/day suggested requirement. High protein foods, such as milk products, eggs, meats, poultry and fresh or canned fish are the best sources of phosphorus. Almonds, string beans, carrots, raisins and cucumbers are other good sources.

Magnesium

Magnesium helps to move nutrients in and out of cells and maintain normal muscle. It also serves important functions related to nerves and bones as well as for many other body systems. Good sources of magnesium are fish, nuts, vegetables, fruits and whole grains.

North American diets are generally sufficient in magnesium. Recommended intake for men and women is 200-400 mg/day. Magnesium supplementation is generally unnecessary, but may be recommended by a healthcare professional for individuals with low magnesium levels caused by poor absorption or intestinal diseases. Magnesium is sometimes combined in calcium supplements, which can be helpful when such supplements cause constipation

Zinc

Zinc can reduce calcium absorption, which is not good for bones. However, with adequate calcium intake of 1,200 mg/day, additional zinc should not have any negative impact on calcium absorption. There are no significant clinical studies proving or refuting the use of zinc to help strengthen bones and reduce fractures. Therefore, there is no reason to recommend supplementation with zinc for the purposes of improving bone health unless a specific zinc deficiency has been diagnosed.

Chapter 5 Key Points

- Calcium from the food you eat is best.
- Recommended total dietary and supplemental calcium intake for adults over 50 is 1,200 mg/day.
- Talk with your pharmacist about ways to manage constipation if you are taking supplemental calcium.
- There are many easy ways to increase your dietary calcium such as substituting cow milk or soy beverage for water when cooking or adding cheese, soy beans or other kinds of beans to a recipe.
- Calculate your daily dietary and supplemental calcium intake at least once a year and compare to recommended daily calcium intake.
- Too much calcium from supplements may be harmful.
- Calcium alone cannot prevent osteoporosis or restore bone health.
- If you do not meet the recommended calcium intake through diet alone, adjust your diet or add a calcium supplement.
- There are many options for calcium supplements if you need one. Choose one that suits you best.
- Vitamin D is necessary for the absorption of calcium and prevention of osteoporosis.
- Many people are deficient in vitamin D.

- Recommended vitamin D intake for healthy adults over 50 is 800-2,000 IU/day; 400-1,000 IU/day for healthy adults 19-50.
- Few foods naturally provide enough vitamin D.
- Daily sunshine exposure of 15-20 minutes with maximum skin exposure and no sunscreen can provide your daily dose of vitamin D. However, be aware of any personal risk you might have to skin cancer. Check with your health care professional.
- Depending on age, vitamin D supplementation of 400-2,000 IU/day may be beneficial as a routine supplement, particularly for people living in cold climates or where there is not enough sunshine.
- Vitamins A and K, phosphorous and protein are all important for bone metabolism, but should be provided in adequate amounts in a healthy, well-balanced diet.
- Vitamin A supplementation may increase health risks if taken in excess.

The Importance of Exercise and Safe Movement

Weight-bearing, resistance (strength) and balance exercises help reduce the risk of osteoporosis, falls and fractures.

The importance of physical activity on bone health is well recognized. Physical activity helps to improve balance, strength, agility and flexibility. Studies show that a person who is inactive or immobilized for a period of time will lose bone. Immobility from lower extremity fractures or surgery is common.

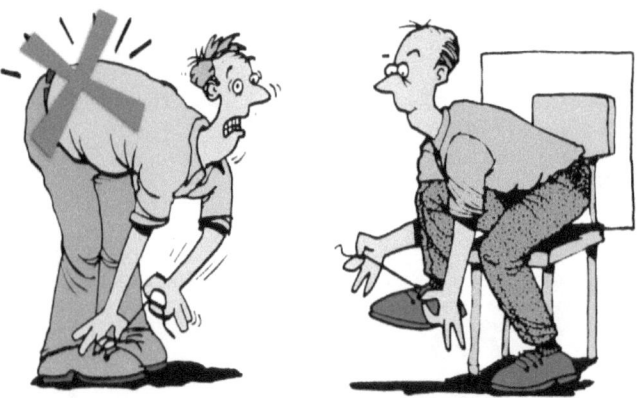

Physical activity is categorized as:
- *non-weight-bearing activities, such as swimming and bicycling*
- *weight-bearing activities, such as Tai Chi, walking, jumping, running and tennis*

Weight-bearing activities transmit weight through the bone. This promotes bone formation and a healthy skeleton. To increase bone density, weight-bearing activities are preferred over non-weight-bearing activities as they usually have more impact on muscle strengthening, balance and improved bone health.

TRAINING EXERCISES

A training program usually comprises various types of exercises to achieve a targeted goal. Types of training exercises include:

Resistance Training

Resistance (strength) training improves or maintains muscular fitness by exercising muscles against an external resistance. The external resistance can be your own body weight or any object that causes the muscles to contract such as training weights, soup cans or elastic tubing.

Balance Training

Balance training helps you to increase the body's agility and thereby reduce your risk of falling. You can include balance training in daily living activities such as balancing on one leg while standing in a grocery line up or at the sink while washing dishes.

Aerobic Training

Aerobic training improves cardiovascular (heart) and lung fitness and, thereby, the body's use of oxygen.

Posture Training

Posture training supports the spine and can help to improve any breathing dysfunction that leads to more rapid shallow, breaths. By improving your posture, you reduce the tightening of the muscles in the chest area, which in turn enables you to take deeper, longer breaths. Better posture and better breathing can improve your walking speed and ability to move more efficiently and safely.

The types and intensity of exercises you choose should match your current health status, ability and tolerance. If you have, or are at risk of developing osteoporosis, then include weight-bearing exercises, which incorporate resistance training to improve strength, and balance training to prevent falls. An aerobic portion of the program may be added if appropriate. For people already in an aerobic or cardiovascular exercise program, consider doing the resistance and balance training before your cardio exercises, when you are less fatigued.

Stretching will also help you maintain and improve your agility and flexibility. This is important to help prevent falls and help you recover if you lose your balance. Many stretching exercises can become resistance exercises by properly adding an external force, such as free weights or exercise bands.

CHOOSING THE APPROPRIATE EXERCISES

10-Year Fracture risk	Appropriate Exercises*
Low	Balance and strengthening or resistance exercises along with an aerobic program
Moderate	Weight-bearing, balance and strengthening, and resistance exercises. Consultation with a physical therapist specializing in osteoporosis is recommended.
High	Consult with a physical therapist specializing in osteoporosis.

* Giangregorio LM, Papaioannou A, Macintyre NJ, et al. Too Fit to Fracture: Exercise recommendations for individuals with osteoporosis or osteoporotic vertebral fracture. *Osteoporosis Int.* 2014 Mar;25(3):821-35. doi: 10.1007/s00198-013-2523-2. Epub 2013 Nov 27

Consider your health status and fracture risk based on your bone mineral density, 10-year risk of fracture, along with your assessment of risk factors for osteoporosis and fracture. Based on your gender, age, health status and current fracture risk assessment, determine if you are at a low, moderate or high risk of fracture.

Choose an exercise program that is right for your body and health status. Consult first with a physical therapist who is experienced in osteoporosis and give consideration to: the proper type of exercises for you; how often you should do them; and how many repetitions you should do. Contact your national or local osteoporosis organizations for certified programs in your community and how to find qualified physical therapists and/or trainers.

If you have not exercised in a while, start out cautiously. As your endurance improves, slowly increase the number of repetitions and resistance to the exercises.

Eventually, increase the variety of exercises. Exercise programs should include stretching for flexibility, muscle-strengthening or resistance training to improve strength and balance training to prevent falls.

Problems with the heart, lungs, joints or other pre-existing conditions may prevent you from doing certain exercises. People with arthritis may find some weight-bearing exercises too painful or difficult. Exercising in water may be an alternative.

WALK, WALK, WALK

Walking is a low force weight-bearing exercise that has a number of health benefits, especially when done at a brisk pace. Walking provides cardio exercise that improves the heart and consumes calories to fight obesity and diabetes. Walking improves mental health, reduces depression, increases self-esteem and improves sleep quality. It increases muscle tone, strength and stamina that will help improve your balance and reduce your risk of falling.

When walking, notice your posture, foot motion, stride, arm movement, breathing and walking speed. Make sure you are getting enough foot and ankle support from your shoes. You might want to ask your healthcare professional to assess your balance and gait. Consider whether your balance, vision, hearing or joints are impaired or compromised. As with any activity, you want to be safe while you walk.

To start a walking program, plan to walk at least three times a week. Fifteen to 30 minutes/session is generally a good start. Start walking slowly and then increase intensity over time. You should not feel discomfort or stiffness after the first week. Be aware of your posture and gait as you walk. Look straight ahead, use your stomach muscles to tuck your tummy in, swing your arms gently and breathe as you move forward.

To improve your cardio, some experts suggest walking 5-6 times a week and include weight training three times a week.

Nordic Walking

Walking poles are sometimes used to increase the intensity of the workout. Nordic walking, also known as urban poling, is a whole-body activity that uses muscles in the shoulders, neck, back and arms as well as the lower half of the body, while reducing the impact on hips and knees during the workout. Nordic walking helps strengthen core muscles and improve posture, coordination and fluid movement.

Before incorporating this type of walking into your exercise routine, know your risk level of fracture and discuss the benefits and risks with your healthcare professional, physical therapist or trainer. Be sure you have the right equipment and instruction. There are some contraindications to using poles, so this type of walking may not be for everyone (e.g., people who are not fully weight-bearing or not able to grip). Certified instructors should be sought to help you move safely and gain the maximum benefit for your efforts.

INTIMACY AND SAFE MOVEMENT

Healthy intimate relationships are an important part of living and one's quality of life. Broadly defined, intimacy is a close familial, personal or emotional relationship. More narrowly defined, intimacy is a physical relationship, usually referring to as sexual expression. Both are correct. The American Occupational Therapy Association has categorized sexual expression as an activity of daily living.

If you engage in a physical relationship, be aware that weak bones may be prone to fracture due to over exertion. However, having low bone density doesn't mean you should avoid sex or that big intimate hug. Intimacy and sex are important elements of human relationships. Do not let fear impact this important part of your life.

Some patients and their partners find the topic difficult to discuss. Good relationships begin with honest communication. If you are not able to start this conversation with your partner, talk to your doctor or ask for a referral to an expert in this field. They can provide information, resources, adaptations and encouragement to find resolutions to your situation.

EXERCISE CONSIDERATIONS AND SAFE MOVEMENT

Be Safe, Move Properly

Be sure you know your own risk of osteoporosis and fracture before beginning any exercise program.

- *Remember to move gently.*
- *If you are at moderate to high risk of osteoporosis, avoid jarring and impact activities. Be aware of your movement and how it impacts your bones.*
- *Learn how to bend and lift correctly.*
- *Keep your back straight and knees bent when you exercise or undertake daily activities such as picking up a child, loading a dishwasher, looking over your shoulder and lifting items from your trunk.*
- *Avoid rounding and twisting your spine.*

If in doubt about an exercise, check it out with an exercise specialist. If you experience pain or discomfort when doing an exercise, stop the exercise immediately and speak with your healthcare professional or trainer. If you are at risk of breaking a bone, be sure you have an instructor qualified in bone health and exercise.

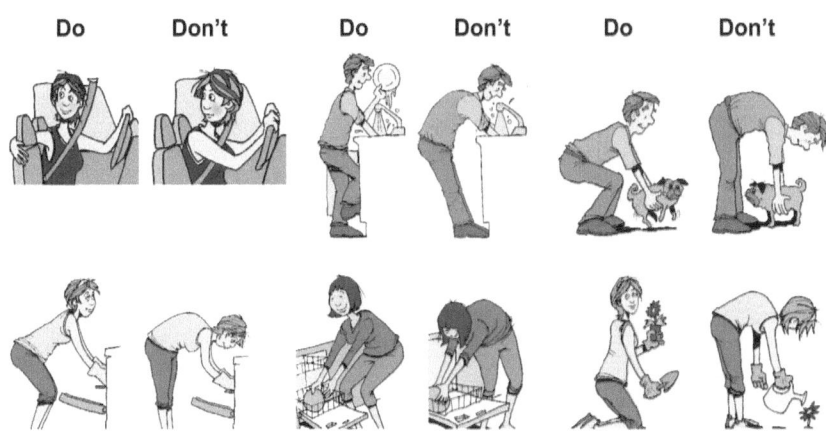

Adapted from American Bone Health's *Doing It Right and Prevent Fractures*

Plan Ahead

No exercise is safe if you injure yourself while doing it. Be careful. Make exercise a routine – commit to a time of day to exercise. The benefits of exercise outweigh the inconvenience. Keep a record of your progress by recording how you feel after each workout. To keep it interesting and to work different muscles, choose a few different exercises each week.

Breathe

Muscles require oxygen to work. Regular, rhythmical breathing as you exercise will help to reduce the internal pressure in your body and allow oxygen to get to the body tissues as it should. During an exercise, breathe out during the exertion phase and breathe in as you relax. Breathe deeply from your diaphragm. Place your hands on your lower ribs and feel them expand and contract as you breathe.

Repetitions

After repeating each exercise three times, remember to completely relax. Relaxing between exercises allows your muscles to gain the full benefit of the exercise. Slowly increase the number of repetitions. If your healthcare professional agrees, try adding one repetition per day to a maximum of 10-12 repetitions working up to two and eventually three complete sets of 10-12 repetitions. Typically, it is recommended that you work up to exercising 30 minute/day, 5 days/week or more depending on your program.

Posture

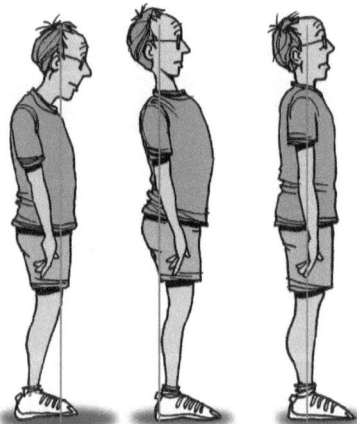

Correct posture, as shown on the right, for a naturally fit person is when the body is in its optimal position with the chin pulled in, the chest up, the lower back arched backward and the abdominal or core muscles pulled in tight to support the lower back. Look straight ahead not down when walking. By stretching and strengthening specific muscle groups, posture can be improved. Work with a physical therapist or trainer to identify and strengthen these muscle groups.

Strong back and abdominal muscles will support the spine and help with correct posture. By maintaining correct posture, you will avoid putting undue stress on your spine. A correct posture will also help promote deep, easier breathing and efficient food digestion. Correct posture, whether sitting, standing or lying down, is important if the muscles and the entire body are to function properly. Posture and how the parts of your body align with each other to move will influence your gait.

Gait

Gait refers to your manner of walking. A normal gait requires a series of smooth, rhythmic movements from initiation to completion of several steps. Muscles and joints line up and coordinate to move properly so that no part of the body is over stressed. Many people do not think about how they move. Be aware of your posture, your foot motion as your heel strikes the ground and roles through the step to push off from your toe.

If you have a problem, such as a sore toe, knee or hip, you do not want to put all your weight on that leg and typically you limp. This inefficient movement as you walk can affect your balance, which in turn increases your risk of falling. An injury, pain from a fracture or surgery, some diseases such as Parkinson's disease, or even poor fitting shoes may cause a limp, shuffle or shaking resulting in a poor gait.

Studies show that gait problems are a major cause of walking difficulties as we get older. Check your gait with your healthcare professional or physical therapist. Once you are aware of a gait problem, you can often remedy the problem through exercise, shoe adjustments or walking support.

Chapter 6 Key Points

- Exercise is good for the whole body.

- Tai Chi is an effective exercise to improve posture and balance.

- The focus for exercise is to build stronger bones and improve strength and balance to prevent falls and fractures.

- The type and amount of exercise you choose should match your health status. Talk with your healthcare professional to determine your health status.

- Walking 15-30 minutes, 3 times/ week is generally a good start to an exercise program.

- Exercising at least 30 minutes/day, 5 days/week or more is recommended for most individuals.

- Plan ahead and make regular exercise a priority.

- Weight-bearing, resistance (strength) and balance exercises help to reduce the risk of osteoporosis and falls.

- When exercising, consider the benefits of safe movements, breathing, number of repetitions and proper posture.

- Check your posture and gait.

CHAPTER 7

Assessing Your Bone Health

Even if you are doing everything right to maintain healthy bones, you can still be susceptible to osteoporosis and fractures. A proper clinical evaluation of your bone health includes an assessment of your bone density, bone quality and blood chemistry.

Osteoporosis-related fractures cause substantial disability, loss of independence, low self-esteem and even death among post-menopausal women and older men. Equally devastating is that many younger women and men with bone loss go under recognized and under treated.

Bone strength comes from the combination of a bone's:

- *quality (architecture or structure)*
- *density (mass: how thick or thin)*
- *ability to repair and develop through remodeling (effected by the mechanics of weight-bearing exercises to stimulate bone remodeling, hormones, nutrition and aging)*

Bone strength is important in determining risk of fracture. A bone is like a stool that you sit on. If any part starts to progressively weaken, the stool will not be as strong as it once was and is more likely to break.

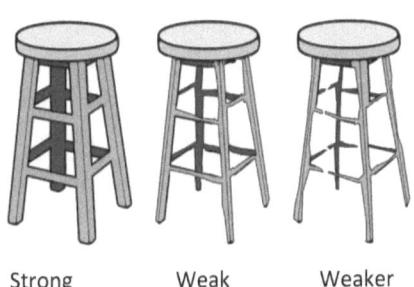

Strong   Weak   Weaker

We know our bones naturally get weaker as we age. Many fractures occur in women and men who have normal or low (osteopenia) bone mineral density rather than osteoporosis. To reduce the risk of fractures due to weak bones, it is imperative that our bone health be regularly assessed as we age.

Remember in the introduction of this book, we asked "Are you at risk?" and showed you the F3D3 tool for quick fracture risk assessment to determine the need for further clinical evaluation. This is a good starting point for identifying risk factors for osteoporosis and future fractures. If you are at risk, then further clinical evaluation by your healthcare professional is required.

Your healthcare professional will review medications you are taking that might cause bone loss and will consider your age, gender and any other health conditions that could affect your bone health. Individuals with osteoporosis-related hip or spine fractures are considered high risk.

After considering the risk factors, you may require a bone mineral density (BMD) test and a 10-year fracture risk assessment using a fracture risk assessment tool such as FRAX. Your healthcare professional may also order a spinal radiography to look for spine fractures and lab tests to rule out secondary osteoporosis. Blood and urine tests, for example, can identify possible causes of bone loss. Once this information is gathered, your healthcare professional will work with you to identify the best treatments to maintain and improve your bone health.

Jill's Story: Assessment Tools

Jill, 44, was encouraged by her older sister to talk with her doctor about her bone health. Jill has no risk factors for osteoporosis other than she has had a number of kidney stones, which she passed. A condition called hyperparathyroidism, which affects about 1 in 1,000 people, is associated with kidney stones and osteoporosis. The doctor suggested Jill have a bone mineral density test. Jill was surprised when the results showed a T-score of her lumbar spine as -4.2 SD (osteoporosis) and her hip as -2.3 SD (low).

Her doctor ordered blood tests to rule out secondary causes of bone loss. The blood tests included measuring serum calcium and parathyroid hormone, which confirmed Jill has hyperparathyroidism. A surgeon recommended a simple operation to remove her parathyroid glands which are pea sized glands in the front of the neck. Jill's bone density should then improve over the next few yeas.

BONE MINERAL DENSITY (BMD) TESTING

A BMD test is a non-invasive procedure that measures the amount of bone material in a defined area of bone. If you have low bone density, you are at a higher risk of a fracture from a fall.

ISCD Indicators for BMD Testing

The International Society for Clinical Densitometry (ISCD) developed the following indicators to determine when a BMD test is necessary:

- *post-menopausal women 65 and older; men 70 and older*
- *post-menopausal women under 65 and men under 70 with clinical risk factors for fracture, such as:*
    - *low body weight*
    - *prior fracture*
    - *high-risk medication use*
    - *disease or condition associated with bone loss*
- *women discontinuing estrogen if they meet the indications in guidelines*
- *frail (weak) patients*
- *peoples with secondary risk factors, including:*
    - *disease or condition associated with low bone density or bone loss (e.g., anorexia, adrenal insufficiency, celiac disease, RA)*
    - *taking medications associated with low bone density or bone loss (e.g., glucocorticoids, anticonvulsants)*
    - *prescribed pharmacologic therapy at the beginning of treatment and to monitor treatment effect over time*
- *individuals at risk of falling, including those:*
    - *not receiving therapy for whom evidence of bone loss would lead to treatment*
    - *with a history of falls in the past year*

- *with risk factors related to aging, disease, medications, environmental factors, poor posture and balance*
- *people who have experienced significant height loss*

Most countries have developed their own protocols similar to the ISCD guidelines for ordering a BMD test. Check with your healthcare professional to see if you should have a BMD test.

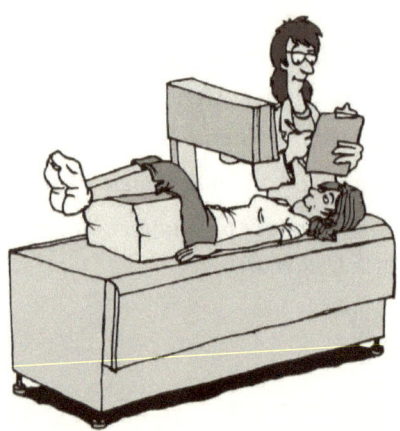

Dual-energy X-ray absorptiometry (DXA)

Bone mineral density is most commonly done using dual-energy X-ray absorptiometry (DXA). The results are reported as a T-score or a Z-score. Typically, a BMD test using DXA does not show bone structure or architecture.

T-Scores

A T-score is the number of standard deviations (SD) that your bone density is above or below what would be expected in the average person of the same gender at age 30.

What does your DXA T-score mean?

Bone Mass	T-Score
Normal	-1 to +2 SD
Low (Osteopenia)	-1 to -2.4 SD
Osteoporosis	-2.5 SD or lower

For each SD reduction in BMD, your risk of fracture doubles:

- **Normal:** *You have up to 10% less bone than the average 30-year-old of the same gender. BMD decreases as we age, so the risk of fracture is considered low.*

- **Low (osteopenia):** *You have up to 25% less bone than the average 30-year-old of the same gender and are at four times greater risk of fracture than the average young adult.*

- **Osteoporosis:** *You have at least 25% less bone than the average 30-year-old of the same gender and are at eight times greater risk of fracture compared to that of an average young adult.*

Although tests other than a DXA can produce T-scores, they do not equate with DXA T-scores and can, therefore, be misleading. It is a good idea whenever necessary, to be retested using the same technology and preferably the same machine so that correct comparisons can be made.

Z-Scores

For most pre-menopausal women and for men, a BMD test will be reported as a Z-score. Z-scores cannot be compared to T-scores. A Z-score is matched to an average person your own age and is useful where enough data exist for comparison. A T-score is generally thought to be the better method of reporting for post-menopausal women.

Many factors go into properly measuring and interpreting a BMD test. Therefore, your BMD should be measured at a reliable clinic with a good quality control program. Ask if the technologists and physicians have specific education and certification in bone densitometry.

Chapter 7 Key Points

- BMD testing should be done to clarify fracture risk.
- DXA is the most common test for measuring bone density.
- If you feel you are at risk of a fracture, have a proper clinical assessment done by your healthcare professional.
- 20% of older patients with fracture have normal or low BMD score (T-Score above -2.5 SD).

- It is your right to ask your technologist about the clinic's policy on machine maintenance and the staff's continuing education. An inaccurate BMD is of no use.

- A T-score is generally for post-menopausal woman. It compares a person's bone density with that of a 30-year old.

- A Z-score is used for pre-menopausal women and for men. It is matched to an average person your own age and is useful when enough data exists for a comparison.

Assessing Your Risk of Fracture

Your 10-year fracture risk can be estimated using the web-based FRAX tool or other fracture assessment tool available in your country.

In addition to BMD testing, other factors need to be considered in order to determine your fracture risk. These include aging, history of falling and previous fractures, family history, diet and lifestyle, disease and medications. Fracture risk assessment tools, such FRAX, evaluate a person's risk of breaking a bone in the future. Unlike a BMD test that requires a machine to measure bone density, FRAX enables you to do your own risk assessment, which you can then review with your healthcare professional.

FRAX, which is freely available online, is the most common international 10-year fracture risk assessment tool. In North America, other assessment tools are sometimes used. These are:

- *FORE FRC, Foundation of Osteoporosis Research and Education's Fracture Risk Calculator. This web-based questionnaire relies on American data and is used only in the United States. It assesses 10-year risk of any one of four fractures (hip, wrist, humerus and spine) and hip fractures for adults over age 45.*

- *CAROC Fracture Risk Assessment developed by the Canadian Association of Radiologists and Osteoporosis Canada uses separate graphs for women and men to assess a person's 10-year risk of fracture. It is based on a Canadian database and is used only in Canada. A T-score for the femoral neck is required to complete the evaluation.*

As with FRAX, FORE FRC and CAROC can be used for patients who have not received any prescription osteoporosis therapies. Both are visual charts that are freely available online. For most people, the results of these two assessment tools will be the same as FRAX. Therefore, which tool to use will be a matter of personal preference by your healthcare professional in the U.S. or Canada. In this chapter we will discuss assessing your fracture risk in more detail using FRAX.

FRAX

FRAX is designed for people in different countries and different ethnic backgrounds. It can be used with or without a BMD test result. It can be used by men and women between the ages of 40 and 90 who have not previously been treated for osteoporosis.

FRAX uses clinical risk factors, bone mineral density and country-specific fracture and mortality data to identify your probability of a hip or major osteoporotic fracture in the next 10 years. If you have had a BMD test prior to completing the FRAX questionnaire, you will be asked for your T-score. If you also received a trabecular bone score (TBS) as part of the BMD test, you will be asked for this as well. Not all BMD machines can produce a TBS. Nevertheless, you can still obtain 10-year fracture risk assessments without it.

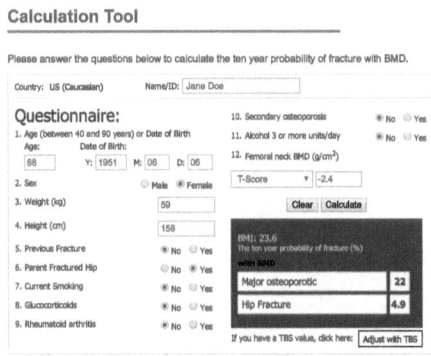

Once you have answered the questions, click the calculate button to see your 10-year probability of a major osteoporotic fracture and hip fracture. If your percentage risk of a major osteoporotic fracture is less than 10%, you are considered at low risk.

10-YEAR FRACTURE PROBABILITY CALCULATED AS A PERCENTAGE

Below 10%	Low Risk: You do not need prescribed therapy for osteoporosis. However, lifestyle changes may be implemented to reduce risk of fracture.
10-20%	Moderate Risk: Further assessment (including BMD test) is required to determine if prescribed therapy is necessary. Further lifestyle changes may be required to reduce risk of fracture.
Higher than 20%	High Risk: Requires prescribed therapy. Lifestyle should be reviewed and changes made as required to reduce risk of fracture.

Most experts recommend if your risk is less than 10%, then preventative non-medication measures should continue. Ten to 20% is considered moderate risk and, depending on your health status and lifestyle choices, consider additional measures that would help to reduce or minimize risk with non-medication measures. If there is a secondary cause of bone loss, medication may be necessary. If your risk is greater than 20%, you are considered to be at high risk and medication is usually recommended. Discuss your risk with your healthcare professional and together identify the best way you can reduce your risk of a future fracture.

For hip fracture risk, if you're percentage risk is equal to or greater than 3%, then you are considered at high risk and should discuss your results, medications and other treatment options with your healthcare professional.

Factors not included in the FRAX questionnaire may also be contributing to your probability of fracturing a bone in the future. Before making treatment recommendations, your healthcare professional will use experienced clinical judgement while considering other factors, such as your history of falls, number of previous fractures, vitamin D levels, and specific secondary causes of bone loss.

Chapter 8 Key Points

- If you break a bone through normal movements or a low energy fall, you likely have osteoporosis. Discuss with your healthcare professional about having a proper risk assessment for osteoporosis and how you can reduce your risk of future fractures.

- Your 10-year fracture risk can be estimated by using the online-based FRAX tool or the FORE Fracture Risk Calculator in the U.S or the CAROC tool in Canada.

- Fracture risk assessment can help you to identify your best treatment plan.

- Fracture risk assessment tools are meant to be accurate for certain age groups who have not taken any prescription osteoporosis medications (past or present). Experts can often adapt the results as needed.

- Interpretation of your fracture risk should be discussed with your healthcare professional if it falls in the moderate- or high-risk category.

- If you are already on treatment, discuss your future fracture risk with your healthcare professional.

Medical Treatment

The goal of medication therapy is to reduce fracture risk by preventing further bone loss and promoting strong bones.

Although some of us prefer not to take medication, some medication may be necessary to help us enjoy the quality of life we desire. While osteoporosis can often be managed through a healthy lifestyle, people with severe osteoporosis are more likely to decide to take medication after a fracture has occurred. If you are at an early stage of osteoporosis with mild to moderate bone loss and no fractures, you might want to discuss your options of whether or not to take a prescribed medication with your healthcare professional.

Choosing the right medication can be a challenge as different medications provide different benefits and, in some cases, side-effects. The main purpose for taking a medication is prevent future fractures. Some medications have a greater impact on the spine while others also impact the hip.

In this chapter, we will review how drug therapies work, treatment options and the benefits and risks of taking prescribed medications.

HOW MEDICATION THERAPY WORKS

When considering a medication's mechanism of action, or how it works, we look at the way it produces an effect on the body. Most medications can be administered through different routes, including:

- *taking pills orally (daily, weekly or monthly)*
- *infusions or intravenous therapy (every three months or once yearly)*
- *subcutaneous (just below the skin) injections (once daily or monthly or every six months)*

Not all medications are available in all forms. Work with your healthcare professional to find the medication that is most effective and affordable for you and best suits your lifestyle. Research shows that people are more likely to take their medication as prescribed if they have agreed to the method and frequency of administration.

Medications used to reduce the risk of future fractures fall under several general categories:

- *Antiresorptive medications slow down bone removal by inhibiting the osteoclast cells.*
- *Anabolic medications assist in bone formation or building by stimulating the osteoblast cells to speed up bone formation.*
- *RANK Ligand (RANKL) inhibition uses a human antibody that binds to RANKL and inhibits the RANKL pathway. RANKL is a protein in the body that stimulates cells to become osteoclast (bone removal) cells. It has an antiresorptive mechanism of action with the added benefit of having a more direct way to slow bone breakdown.*
- *Sclerostin inhibition uses a human antibody that works by interfering with the activity of the protein sclerostin and, as a result, has a dual effect on bone by increasing bone formation and decreasing bone breakdown*

Medication treatments used to reduce the risk of future fractures are:

- *bisphosphonates*
- *denosumab*
- *selective estrogen receptor modulators (SERMs)*
- *parathyroid hormone therapy*
- *hormone therapy*
- *romosozumab*

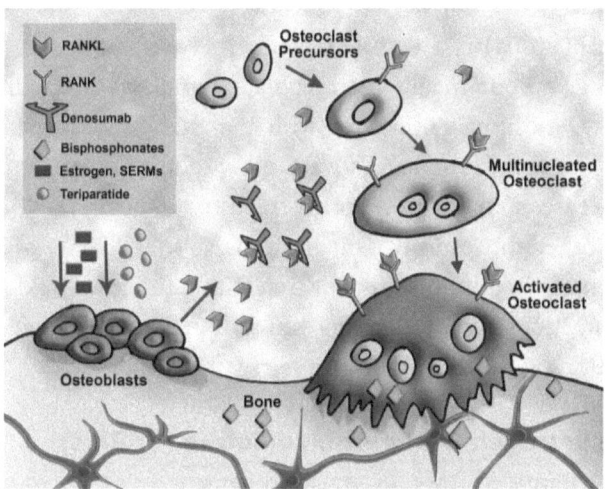

Medication Treatments and How They Work

Bisphosphonates

Bisphosphonates are the most widely used class of antiresorptive medication for reducing the risk of future fractures. They slow down bone removal by interfering with osteoclast (bone removal) cells and enabling the osteoblast (bone building) cells to work more effectively. By slowing down the action that removes bone material, bone thinning or loss is slowed.

Because bisphosphonates have slightly differing characteristics, one bisphosphonate may be more effective than another for a particular therapy. Bisphosphonates approved for the treatment of osteoporosis in Canada and the United States are: alendronate (Fosamax, Fosavance), risedronate (Actonel, Actonel with calcium, Actonel DR, Atelvia) and zoledronic acid (Reclast, Aclasta). The United States also has ibandronate (Boniva). While other bisphosphonates are available in the United States and Canada, they have not been approved for use reducing fracture risk.

Bisphosphonate medications are taken orally, with the exception of zoledronic acid (Reclast, Aclasta), which is administered intravenously once a year. When taking an oral bisphosphonate, it is important to follow specific directions so that the medication is allowed to work properly with minimal side-effects. Calcium interferes with the absorption of bisphosphonates and should not be consumed two hours before or after taking a bisphosphonate.

Denosumab

Denosumab (Prolia) is a RANK Ligand (RANKL) inhibitor (sometimes referred to as a bone metabolism regulator) and has effects like an anti-resorptive. Denosumab interferes with the RANKL's normal actions of stimulating osteoclast (bone removal) cells. Studies have shown that denosumab decreases spinal, hip and other fractures and increases bone density more than other antiresorptive medications.

Denosumab is administered by injection under the skin every six months. Injections can be done by you at home after receiving guidance and education on the technique by a nurse or pharmacist.

Selective Estrogen Receptor Modulators (SERMs)

Despite the name, SERMs are not estrogens; they are a compound that interacts with the body's tissues. Sometimes the SERM acts like estrogen (e.g., in the bones) and at other times, it has the effect of blocking estrogen (e.g., in the uterus and breast). Experts find that the SERM Raloxifene, a single dose tablet taken daily, is most appropriate for active women who are recently post-menopause, generally in their early sixties, as it has been shown to reduce spine fractures for women at low risk of fracture. A word of caution, post-menopausal symptoms, such as hot flashes (flushes) and other vasomotor symptoms, are not effectively managed by Raloxifene and may get worse.

Bazedoxifene and conjugated estrogens is a combination SERM medication approved for women during peri-menopausal years to treat moderate to severe menopausal symptoms. Taken daily as a single dose tablet, it is generally recommended that treatments be limited to women under 60 years of age or until menopausal symptoms are no longer an issue.

Once either of these medications is stopped, its bone benefit will end. A proper fracture risk assessment should be done to determine the best course of treatment going forward.

Parathyroid Hormone Therapy

Teriparatide (Forteo) is a synthetic form of the naturally occurring parathyroid hormone (PTH). It is a well-established osteoporosis treatment that directly impacts the bone building or the anabolic part of the bone remodeling process. Teriparatide is approved for the treatment in post-menopausal women, for men at high risk for fracture and for glucocorticoid-induced osteoporosis.

Abaloparatide (Tymlos), a human parathyroid hormone-related protein, is a bone building treatment, indicated for post-menopausal women with osteoporosis at high risk for fracture or who have failed on other treatments.

Both treatments are administered once a day by injection under the skin and should not be used for more than 24 consecutive months, at which time you will be switched to different therapy, likely an anti-resorptive. Studies have shown both treatments to reduce spinal fractures and other fractures.

Hormone Therapy

Hormone therapy or estrogen/progesterone is often used to treat symptoms of menopause and has the added benefit of increasing bone density and preventing hip and spine fractures. With the advent of other drug therapies, estrogen has been taken off the primary list of osteoporosis treatments in the United States, but it is approved for osteoporosis therapy in Canada, usually when severe menopausal symptoms are also an issue.

Testosterone replacement therapy is a preventive measure for osteoporosis when indicated for men who generally display other hypogonadal symptoms. It is not, however, considered a medical treatment for osteoporosis as there are more effective medical treatments available for bone loss.

Romosozumab

Sclerostin is a protein that regulates bone formation. Romosozumab (Evenity) is an anti-sclerostin dual action mode therapy, designed to work by simultaneously building bone (anabolic action) and, to a lesser extent, slowing bone loss (anti-resorptive action).

It is administered once a month by a healthcare provider for 12 consecutive months. Once completed, continued therapy with an anti-resorptive should be considered. The medication comes with a warning for older adults with a high risk of heart disease or stroke.

Leslie's Story: Rare Events

Leslie, 60, has been on weekly bisphosphonates for five years to reduce her risk of fracture and is doing well. Her dentist suggests that she have a number of implants, but he is reluctant to do any dental work as Leslie might be vulnerable to osteonecrosis of the jaw (ONJ), a rare condition in people being treated with bisphosphonates. ONJ shows up as an area of exposed bone inside the mouth that may or may not be painful. Medical and dental authorities have developed guidelines on how to manage situations like Leslie's.

BENEFIT, RISK AND COST FACTORS

Before going on a medication to reduce the risk of future fractures, consider its benefits as well as its risks and cost. In all cases, the decision to take medication is yours and there are many useful medications to consider. For example, most experts agree that alendronate (Fosamax), risedronate (Actonel) and zoledronic acid (Reclast, Aclasta) are among the most effective bisphosphonates for reducing fractures. These medications can reduce the chances of a fracture by about half or more. In more recent studies, denosumab (Prolia) has been shown to increase bone density to a larger amount than other antiresorptive medications.

SIDE-EFFECTS AND RARE EVENTS

Side-effects and rare events can occur when taking any medication. Side-effects tend to be mild, usually go away in a few days and do not cause long-term damage. Rare events are more serious, but less common. Osteonecrosis of the jaw is one example of a rare event that could be related to long term use of bisphosphonates. While extremely rare, take good care of your teeth. If concerned, talk to your doctor and dentist before starting on a bisphosphonate. Atypical femoral fracture is another extremely rare event related to long term use of bisphosphonates. Constant aching pain in the thigh or groin is an early warning sign that should be met with a visit to your doctor.

Some side-effects can be eliminated by taking precautions to avoid anything that may make you more susceptible to that side effect. For example, side-effects related to the IV infusion of zoledronic acid can be minimized by drinking plenty of fluids during the day of infusion.

There is always a risk that a devastating, but rare event could occur from taking a medication. Unfortunately, it is not possible to predict when a rare event will occur or who it will affect. Even common, everyday foods have a rare event risk. For example, some people have life-threatening allergic reactions to peanuts or seafood. However, not everyone knows they are allergic.

Examine the potential positive and negative results of taking any medication to prevent the risk of future fractures. Look at how your risk of fracture might progress should you choose not to take the medication. If you were to break a bone, how would your quality of life be affected? Consider your age, gender, diet, activity level and health status. Consider living with a collapsed spine, a curved spine, or broken hip and how that might affect your independence.

After doing your own research and discussing this with your healthcare professional, ask yourself: "Do the benefits of taking or not taking a medication outweigh the short-term and long-term risks of fracture?"

TAKING MEDICATION

If you decide you will benefit from medication, make sure you take it. While this may sound obvious, research shows that only one in four people who are prescribed a medication actually take the medication as they should. Almost half discontinue the medication all together. To be effective, medications must be taken as directed.

The good news is that studies have shown that medications can significantly reduce your risk of a fracture if taken correctly. If you decide it is important for your wellness and quality of life to take the medication, find a medication that matches your lifestyle and is easy for you to remember to take. Then make sure you take the medication as prescribed! If there are issues taking medication, discuss them with your healthcare professional and pharmacist.

Do not let osteoporosis or the fear of breaking a bone take over your life. Use available resources and support to find a healthy way to live a balanced life while managing the disease. Focus on maintaining or improving your health. Focus on your quality of life and wellness rather than the disease.

NON-MEDICAL STRATEGIES TO PROTECT YOUR BONES

Because weak bone puts patients at greater risk of future fractures, emphasis should be placed on strengthening and protecting bones, and preventing the first fracture. Non-pharmacologic strategies to reduce risk of fracture include:

- *adequate intake of calcium, vitamin D and protein*
- *reducing caffeine and dietary sodium to fewer than 2,100 mg/day*
- *physical activity, particularly weight-bearing, strength training and resistance exercises to improve upper and lower body strength and balance*
- *awareness of height loss and propensity to fall*
- *awareness of risk factors associated with aging (e.g., sight, hearing, muscles, gait)*
- *awareness of safe movements for the spine (e.g., lifting, twisting, bending forward)*

Read about Leslie's options for medical treatment in Chapter 10.

Chapter 9 Key Points

- The goal of medication therapy is to reduce fracture risk by preventing further bone loss and promoting strong bones.
- Different medications work in different ways to produce an effect on the body and improve bone density.
- Even while taking prescription medications for osteoporosis, you need to maintain physical exercise and adequate intake of calcium and vitamin D.
- Different medications: slow down osteoclast (bone removal) cells; speed up osteoblasts (bone building) cells; interfere with the action of the protein RANKL, thereby slowing down the tearing down of bone; both build bone and slow bone loss.

- When deciding to take a medication, consider the benefits and risks associated with your health status, lifestyle preferences, risk of osteoporosis and risk of fracture.
- Keep side-effects in perspective. Most go away with time; others may be recurrent. Take steps to minimize the occurrence of side-effects.
- Rare events can be more serious, but much less common

CHAPTER 10

Living with Osteoporosis

Stories

LOW BONE MASS (OSTEOPENIA)

Sandy's recent experience in a research study on bone health has motivated her to follow up with a nurse practitioner at a local community healthcare center. Sandy, a 42-year-old nurse, is fit and active – regularly cycling, hiking, playing tennis and swimming. She eats a healthy diet complemented by supplements and vitamins and has regular monthly periods. She has never smoked, broken a bone or suffered from a significant disease.

The study required a baseline bone mineral density test using a DXA scan. Sandy's T-score was -2.3 SD. While not in the osteoporotic range, her T-score indicates she is in the low bone (osteopenia) density range. Sandy learned that she may have up to 25% less bone than the average 30-year-old female. She was told this could be a warning that she may be at risk of breaking a bone sometime in the next 10 years.

The nurse practitioner explains that because Sandy is still fairly young, her lower than normal bone density may be related to genetics and family history. Sandy remembers her grandmother as a small, elderly lady with hunched over posture, possible due to a curved spine caused by collapsing vertebrae. Sandy does not like milk and seldom drank a glass of milk or ate cheese or yogurt, thus reducing her daily intake of calcium while growing up.

The nurse practitioner reviews Sandy's medical history and orders blood tests. The tests show that Sandy's calcium absorption is fine but her vitamin D level is low.

While Sandy cannot increase her peak bone mass, she can try to slow down her bone loss. The nurse practitioner advises that Sandy does not need medication therapy at this time. However, Sandy could make a couple of changes to her diet and exercise regimen. She recommends that

Sandy consume at least 1,000-1,200 mg/day of calcium through her daily food intake and add 600-1,000 IU/day of vitamin D supplementation. She should be re-checked in a few months to be sure the vitamin D is being absorbed. Sandy should maintain her active lifestyle, but should consider adding strength training to her regimen.

Discussion

Women reach their peak bone mass by about age 20 and men by about age 25. A high peak bone mass is critically important. Bone density then stays stable until the mid-thirties, at which time women and men start to lose bone.

Age-related bone loss occurs at a rate of about 0.5-1% a year. The rate of bone loss increases significantly in women during peri-menopause, which usually starts in a woman's forties, and after menopause at which time a woman's chance of getting osteoporosis increases sharply. However, some younger women experience significant bone loss and even osteoporosis.

Calcium, vitamin D and protein are the main nutrients for maintaining bone health and preventing bone loss. According to National Osteoporosis Foundation guidelines, when determining how much calcium to recommend, assess the amount of calcium being ingested in the diet and top up with supplementation to reach 1,200 mg/day for women over 50 and men over 70 and 1,000 mg for anyone under 50. Osteoporosis Canada guidelines say 1,200 mg for women and men over 50, and 1,000 mg for people aged 19-50. Calcium is best when it comes from food. However, if you need a supplement a single dose of calcium supplement does not need to exceed 500 mg as it may not be adequately absorbed by the body.

Vitamin D promotes calcium absorption in the gut, which helps to maintain blood calcium levels. Unfortunately, many people have low vitamin D levels. Even moderate vitamin D deficiency can affect bone density and structure. Natural vitamin D comes from two main sources: dietary intake and skin exposure to the sun. Supplementation is often needed to achieve required daily intake, especially if you spend a lot of time indoors and have limited skin exposure to the sun. Most experts recommend that adults under 50 need 400-1,000 IU/day of vitamin D and adults over 50 need about 800-2,000 IU/day. Too much vitamin D in the blood, although rare, can be dangerous.

The importance of physical activity on bone health is well recognized. Exercise helps to improve balance, strength, agility and flexibility. Studies show that a person who is inactive or immobile for a period of time will lose bone.

With age, we lose power (ability to generate force quickly) more than strength (amount of force exerted over time). That is, you may have the strength to cross the road before the light changes but you do not have the power to get across the road quickly enough before the light changes.

Even a very active person will still experience some muscle loss. Resistance and weight-bearing activities promote bone density. Weight-bearing exercises and resources include walking, dancing, tennis, jogging, Tai Chi, yoga, Bone Sense and Osteofit. Resistance training improves or maintains fitness by exercising muscles against an external resistance. The external resistance can be one's own body weight, weights or any object that causes the muscles to contract. Resistance training that works on each major muscle done at least twice weekly will build strength and improve balance to protect against falling.

MEN AND OSTEOPOROSIS

Robert, 55, broke his right wrist when he fell rushing across a parking lot. Robert has always had a poor diet and he smokes a pack of cigarettes a day despite having asthma. Treatment for his asthma has included inhaled steroids puffers and frequent short courses of prednisone with flares. His doctor recognizes risk factors for osteoporosis and suggests Robert have a BMD test.

When the BMD DXA shows that Robert has osteoporosis, the doctor suggests tests to rule out secondary causes of the osteoporosis so that treatment options can be decided upon. He recommends that he and Robert do a 10-year fracture assessment using FRAX. He also orders blood tests for Roberts, including total and free testosterone to check for the presence of any medical conditions, such as hypogonadism.

Discussion

Testosterone is the male hormone responsible for secondary sexual features, such as musculature and strength, low voice, a beard and sex drive or libido. It affects many of the body's systems including the brain, heart and skeleton.

Today, we know that osteoporosis not only affects one in three women, but that aging males should also be assessed for osteoporosis and fracture risk. The amount of a man's testosterone declines with age (about 1%/year after age 30). It is estimated that 10% of men over the age of 50 experience symptoms of low testosterone and that one in five men over the age of 50 suffer from low bone density or osteoporosis.

Some medications, such as the steroid prednisone, can cause significant bone loss leading to fractures. Patients should ask if their medication can cause bone loss and be educated to manage medication use properly. They should have good calcium and vitamin D intake. It is important to keep active with a walking program and other weight-bearing, resistance and balance exercises. Ideally, patients like Robert need to get help to stop smoking.

Treatments for secondary causes of bone loss in men may include testosterone replacement therapy if they are hypogonadal (low testosterone). Therapies that include bisphosphonates (alendronate, risedronate, zoledronic acid, denosumab) are proven treatments for men as well as for women. Similarly, teriparatide has been shown to be effective in men with osteoporosis as well as in people who are on prednisone.

SECONDARY OSTEOPOROSIS

Betty, a 55-year-old teacher, has had rheumatoid arthritis for seven years. The disease is moderately active. She had been on low-dose prednisone for many years to control her symptoms. Recently, since her doctor has put her on a biologic medication which she regularly self-injects, Betty has had a dramatic improvement of her arthritis and has stopped taking the prednisone.

However, Betty wonders if she should now go on a medication to prevent further bone loss. Rheumatoid arthritis is commonly associated with bone loss because of active inflammation, decreased physical activity and medications such as prednisone. As her rheumatoid arthritis has been active for seven years and she had been taking prednisone for a few years, Betty already has two significant risk factors for osteoporotic fractures.

To determine if she is prone for fractures in the future, Betty and her doctor do a 10-year fracture risk assessment using FRAX. Betty's earlier DXA test showed that T-score of the hip was fortunately quite low. However, with her rheumatoid arthritis and long-term use of prednisone combined with the fact that her mother had a hip fracture, Betty's 10-year risk of a major osteoporotic fracture is extremely high. To reduce this risk, Betty agrees to go on a medication for five years after which her bone health status will be re-evaluated.

The doctor advises Betty to do regular weight-bearing exercises, ensure that she is getting adequate calcium in her diet and to take a vitamin D supplement. Calcium and vitamin D intake, appropriate exercise programs and lifestyle choices are important in managing secondary osteoporosis.

Discussion

Secondary osteoporosis is when disease, immobility or medication are identified as the cause of the bone loss or a fracture. Secondary osteoporosis remains a challenge to identify and treat as it frequently affects patient populations that are usually not targeted for routine screening for osteoporosis, such as men or pre-menopausal women. Several disease conditions can cause an imbalance in bone resorption and bone formation that result in subsequent bone loss. Rheumatoid arthritis is commonly associated with bone loss because of active inflammation, decreased physical activity and medications such as prednisone.

Due to their effect on bone remodeling, certain medications taken in low dosages over long periods of time can lead to bone loss. Glucocorticoid medications are the most serious cause of medication-induced osteoporosis and subsequent fracture risk. The most common glucocorticoid is prednisone, which is used to treat diseases associated with excessive inflammation. The good news is that recent research suggests that glucocorticoid-induced osteoporosis can be prevented. Since bone loss is most rapid in the first six months of glucocorticoid use, preventive measures should begin immediately if glucocorticoid therapy is expected to go beyond three months.

BMD tests using a DXA scan or other BMD measurement tool should be considered for patients with secondary risk factors, including:

- *long-term immobility associated with a cast, illness or accident*
- *diseases or conditions associated with low bone density or bone loss (e.g., Crohn's disease)*
- *medications associated with low bone density or bone loss (e.g., glucocorticoids)*

As discussed in chapter 7, DXA results are reported as a T-score – the number of standard deviations (SD) above or below the bone density of a healthy 30-year-old of the same gender. A T-score of -2.5 SD or lower means osteoporosis is present and the patient is at a greater risk of fracture.

FRAX is the most commonly used 10-year fracture risk assessment tool. While anyone can complete a FRAX risk assessment online, it is most effective when used in conjunction with a physician or nurse practitioner who understands the significance of the questions asked and can help you determine if treatment is warranted.

MEDICAL TREATMENTS: RISKS AND BENEFITS

Leslie, 60, has been on weekly bisphosphonates for five years to prevent further bone loss and is doing well. On a recent visit, her dentist suggested that she have a number of implants, but he is reluctant to do any dental work as Leslie might be vulnerable to osteonecrosis of the jaw (ONJ), a rare condition in people being treated with bisphosphonates for osteoporosis. ONJ shows up as an area of exposed bone inside the mouth that may or may not be painful.

Current consensus accepts a causal relationship between ONJ and bisphosphonate exposure, but it is unpredictable and rare (0.1%). The strongest association is in patients with cancer (breast, prostate, myeloma) who have been on monthly intravenous bisphosphonates for a year or longer.

Leslie visits her doctor who discusses the benefit of staying on bisphosphonates as it relates to fragility fracture versus the risk going off the medication for awhile. Leslie's doctor and dentist refer to their respective professional guidelines and protocols. They agree that it is reasonable for

Leslie to stop the bisphosphonates for one or two months and then have the dental procedure.

Discussion

Keeping your mouth clean and healthy by regularly brushing your teeth and flossing or cleaning between your teeth is important in protecting yourself against ONJ. However, side-effects and rare events may occur when taking any medication. Unfortunately, it is not possible to predict when a rare event will occur or who it will affect.

Oral bisphosphonates are generally well tolerated when taken properly. However, there can be side-effects and adverse events of bisphosphonates. Some dentists do not feel comfortable performing dental work on a person who is taking a bisphosphonate. Many experts recommend delaying the start of the bisphosphonate therapy until after major dental work has been completed or stopping the bisphosphonate for up to three months prior to major or significant dental procedures, such as tooth extractions or dental implants. Despite this concern, there is evidence that dental implants can be successful in people taking bisphosphonates. More common dental procedures, such as root canals or scaling, so not pose the same concerns.

CHAPTER 11

Resources

The organizations listed on these pages can provide you with additional information about osteoporosis and bone health. Most can be easily found through a search of the internet

---

ILLNESS AND PREVENTION

Centers for Disease Control and Prevention (USA)

1-800-232-4636, cdc.gov

Institute for Safe Medication Practices

(215) 947-7797, consumermedsafety.org

National Institute of Arthritis and Musculoskeletal and Skin Diseases

(301) 495-4484, niams.nih.gov

Public Health agency of Canada

(416) 973-0003, publichealth.gc.ca

OSTEOPOROSIS

Foundation for Osteoporosis Research and Education (FORE)
American Bone Health

(510) 832-2663 or 1-888-266-3015, americanbonehealth.org

National Osteoporosis Foundation

(202) 223-2226 or 1-800-231-4222, nof.org

Canadian Osteoporosis Patient Network (COPN)

(Patient arm of Osteoporosis Canada)
1-800-463-6842, osteoporosis.ca

Osteoporosis Canada

(416) 696-2663 or 1-800-463-6842 (English), osteoporosis.ca

International Osteoporosis Foundation

+41 22 994 0100, iofbonehealth.org

MENOPAUSE
The North American Menopause Society

(440) 442-7550 or 1-800-774-5342, menopause.org

The Society of Obstetricians and Gynaecologists of Canada

(613) 730-4192 or 1-800-561-2416, menopauseandu.ca, sogc.org

NUTRITION
American Dietetic Association

(312) 899-0040 or 1-800-877-1600, eatright.org

Office of Dietary Supplements

(301) 435-2920, ods.od.nih.gov

National Institutes of Health

(301) 435-2920, ods.od.nih.gov

US Department of Agriculture, Center for Nutrition Policy and Promotion

My Pyramid Food Guidance System: 1-888-779-7264 mypyramid.gov

Dietitians of Canada – Find a Dietitian

(416) 596-0857 Find a dietitian: 1-888-901-7776
dietitians.ca/find

Health Canada

1-866-225-0709, hc-sc.gc.ca

Glossary

Anabolic – processes, usually using drugs, that cause bone tissue to build. This may be done by affecting the osteoblast cells and improving bone formation.

Androgen – a substance, such as testosterone, that produces or stimulates the development of male characteristics, such as the hormone testosterone.

Anorexia Nervosa – eating disorder characterized by a fear of becoming obese. It can lead to osteoporosis.

Bisphosphonates – group of drugs used in the treatment of osteoporosis.

Body Mass Index (BMI) – method for assessing body weight in relation to health for most adults. To calculate your BMI, divide your metric weight by your metric height squared. A BMI of 18.5¬24.9 is considered healthy for most adults.

Bone Density – the amount of calcium projected per square centimeter of bone. Also referred to as bone quantity of bone density.

Bone Density Test – an enhanced form of imaging used to measure bone loss. Nuclear imaging helps diagnose and track several types of bone disease. Also referred to as bone densitometry, or dual-energy X-ray absorptiometry (DXA)

Bone Matrix – intracellular (between the cells) substance from which bone is made or develops. It contributes to bone strength.

Bone Mineralization – final stage of bone development that hardens or stiffens bone. Bone matrix produced by osteoblasts mineralizes by the deposits of calcium apatite. The result is new bone.

Bone Mineral Density – average mineral concentration of a section of bone. Synonymous with bone density.

Bone Quality – architecture and microarchitecture of bone.

Bone Quantity – density or mass of bone.

Bone Remodeling – process of bone resorption and formation, which is responsible for renewal of bone.

Calcitonin – hormone produced by the thyroid gland. Calcitonin helps save calcium in the bone. It protects the bone from loss and can be a strong analgesic or pain reliever.

Calcitriol – active hormone form of vitamin D that: promotes the absorption of calcium and phosphorus in the intestines; decreases calcium excretion by the kidneys; and acts along with the parathyroid hormone to maintain bone balance (homeostasis).

Calcium – metallic element found in most living tissues. It is required for bone formation and mineralization, muscle contraction, blood coagulation and the transmission of nerve impulses.

Cortical Bone – compact dense bone that forms the outer shell of all bones.

Cortisol (Cortisone, Prednisone) – hormone secreted by the adrenal glands to regulate the metabolism of fats, carbohydrates and proteins. It also acts as an anti-inflammatory agent.

Dual-Energy X-Ray Absorptiometry (DXA) – method used to measure the amount of bone, usually in the lumbar spine and hip. It is usually done by a machine called a densitometer.

Elemental Calcium – the active portion of a calcium supplement.

Estrogen Therapy – treatment used to correct a deficiency of estrogen, such as after menopause or after the surgical removal of ovaries.

Estrogens – hormones produced by the female sex glands. They are responsible for the development of sexual characteristics in women.

Fat-Soluble Vitamins – able to dissolve in fat and stored in the body tissues.

Femoral neck – the upper thigh bone or area just below the ball of the ball-and-socket hip joint.

Fiber – nutrient found in bran, brown rice, fruit, vegetables and some dairy products. The importance of fiber in the diet cannot be overemphasized.

Fracture – broken bone.

Fragility Fracture – a weak bone at increased risk of fracture from a minor injury that otherwise should not result in a fracture. It is an osteoporosis-related fracture. Occurs spontaneously, such as a fall from a standing height or less, or from a minor injury that otherwise should not fracture normal bone

Fracture Liaison Service – a coordinated service implemented by health-care systems to enhance communication between healthcare professionals to benefit fragility fracture patients by providing a care pathway to identify and treat osteoporosis and prevent a second fracture.

Gait – a person's manor of walking, stride, pace; the way a person carries their body.

Genetics – refers to the number of body traits, such as eye and hair color, height and some diseases, that occur as a result of DNA passed on to you from your parents.

Height Loss – a natural occurrence as we age. A loss of 2.5 inches (6 cm) or greater compared to your historical height loss (the amount of height you have lost since your tallest measurement), or a one-inch (2.5 cm) loss over three years, called prospective height loss, may be cause for concern. To accurately measure your height, first measure your height, then step away and go back and repeat the measurement twice more

Hormone Therapy– treatment used to correct a deficiency of the hor-mones: estrogen, progesterone or testosterone.

Hypogonadism – condition in which the body does not produce enough sex hormone, generally estrogen in women and testosterone in men.

Hysterectomy – surgical removal of the female uterus.

International Units (IU) – measure a drug's potency, not its mass or weight.

Kyphosis – outward curvature of the upper spine caused by the collapse of the vertebrae.

Lactase – intestinal enzyme that breaks down the milk sugar, lactose.

Lactose – a natural sugar found in milk and milk products. lactose Intolerance – occurs when the body cannot produce enough lactase to break down the lactose, resulting in abdominal or digestive tract symptoms.

Lordosis – inward curvature of the lower spine.

Low-Trauma Fracture – low impact fracture or broken bone that occurs from a fall from a standing height or less.

Mechanism of Action – the way a medication exerts an effect on tissue or cells.

Menopause – the moment a woman has no menstrual period after 12 consecutive months.

Metabolism – process whereby the body converts food into living tissue and energy.

Milligram (mg) – a unit of weight equal to one thousandth of a gram.

Mineralization – depositing of minerals in tissues.

Non-Vertebral Fracture – fractures other than those of the spine (back).

Non-Weight-Bearing Exercises – non-impact exercises, such as swimming.

Nutrients – foods that promote life by providing nourishment for growth, repair and metabolism of body tissue.

Osteoblasts – cells that form bone by laying down a matrix that mineralizes.

Osteoclasts – cells involved with the resorption (removal) of bone.

Osteocytes – bone-forming cells entrapped within the bone matrix that help maintain bone as a living tissue.

Osteopenia – occurs when bone mineral density is lower than normal, but not low enough to be considered osteoporosis. Some experts feel this may be a pre-cursor to osteoporosis.

Osteoporotic Vertebral (Spinal) Fracture– a fracture in the spine where bone loss in the spine has caused the vertebrae to become weak and porous to the point the vertebrae eventually collapses or breaks.

Osteoprotegerin (OPG) – part of the body's natural bone tissue defense. It is a protein that blocks RANKL from stimulating bone resorption. oxalates – compounds found in foods, such as beet greens, rhubarb, sorrel, spinach, summer squash, chocolate, cocoa and peanuts, that can interfere with the absorption of calcium.

Parathyroid Hormone – secreted by the parathyroid gland. It promotes bone resorption (removal).

Peak Bone Mass – the point at which your bone building and removal are equal and you have reached your maximum bone density and strength.

Phosphorus – non-metallic element in all living tissue and is involved in most metabolic processes. Phosphorus and calcium are components of bone.

Phytates – phosphorus-containing compounds found in raw, unprocessed foods, such as legumes or outer husks of cereals, bran and oatmeal. They can interfere with the absorption of calcium.

Progesterone – female hormone produced by the ovaries during the second half of the menstrual cycle.

Progestin – hormone that prepares the lining of the uterus for implantation of a fertilized ovum. Synonymous with progesterone.

Progestogen – any natural or synthetic hormonal substance that produces effects similar to those produced by progesterone.

Quantitative Computed Tomography (QCT) Scan – method for measuring bone density that allows direct measurement of a particular area of bone found in the spine. It does not provide T-score compatible with the classification of osteoporosis. radius – the slightly shorter of the two forearm bones. It is found on the thumb side of the forearm and rotates to allow the hand to pivot at the wrist.

RANK (Receptor Activator for Nuclear Factor kB) – protein receptor that controls the maturation of the osteoclast cells it is connected to. When this receptor is activated by RANKL, it stimulates the osteoclast to activate and break down bone.

RANKL (Receptor Activator for Nuclear Factor kB Ligand) – naturally occurring protein in the body that is released by osteoblast cells and acts as the major signal to promote bone removal or resorption.

Resorption – removal of bone by osteoclasts.

Rheumatoid Arthritis – a chronic inflammatory disease mainly of the joints. Inflammation in other body organs and tissues can also occur. Joints are swollen, tender, warm and stiff and have limited movement.

Sex Hormone Binding Globulin (SHBG) – a protein made by your liver and then carried throughout the body. SHBG controls the amount of testosterone that your body tissues can use.

Testosterone – the principle androgen or male sex hormone produced in the gonads. It is responsible for masculine characteristics. It is also produced by the adrenal cortex of both men and women. It affects several tissues in the body. testosterone replacement therapy – treatment to correct a deficiency of testosterone, such as for men who are hypogonadal.

Thyroid Hormones – secreted by the thyroid gland that regulate metabolism.

Trabecular Bone – spongy, porous, less dense bone.

Trabecular Bone Score (TBS) – non-invasive technology derived from DXA image using software to look at the distribution of bone density in the DXA examination of the lumbar spine.

Trauma – physical injury cause by an external force.

Ultrasound (when used to look at osteoporosis) – a procedure that bounces sound waves through the wrist or heel to measure the bone density in that area. It is used as a screening test for osteoporosis, but further research is needed to establish its reliability for other uses. The T-score derived from ultrasound machines do not fit in to the WHO classification.

Vertebra – the singular of vertebrae. There are seven cervical vertebrae, 12 thoracic vertebrae, five lumbar vertebrae, five sacral (fused to form one bone) vertebrae, and four coccygeal (fused to form one coccyx) vertebrae.

Vitamin A – fat-soluble vitamin essential for normal growth and development. It is formed within the body from the yellow pigment of plants. The daily requirement for adults is about 1,000mg. Retinol is the form of vitamin A found in mammals.

Vitamin D– fat-soluble vitamin provided in the diet, manufactured by the action of sunlight on skin, or taken as a supplement. It is converted in the liver and kidney to calcitriol – a hormone that helps in the absorption of calcium and phosphorus.

Vitamin K – fat-soluble vitamin found in most green vegetables. It plays a role in bone metabolism and blood clotting.

Weight-Bearing Exercises – exercises in which weight is applied directly to the bone against the force of gravity. Examples are walking, dancing or climbing stairs. Weight-bearing exercises are necessary in order to maintain healthy bones.

About the Authors

Gwen Ellert, MEd, BScN

A nurse consultant and educator, Gwen authored and published the best-selling *The Arthritis Exercise Book*, accompanied by workshops and videos, aimed at helping people with arthritis live their lives to the maximum. Following the success of *The Arthritis Exercise Book*, she co-wrote two editions of *The Osteoporosis Book* with rheumatologist Dr. John Wade, which were endorsed by Osteoporosis Canada, and the third and fourth editions retitled *The Osteoporosis Book: Bone Health* with Dr. Wade and pharmacist Dr. Alan Low. It is currently being used in the American Bone Health Peer Educator Program. Her nursing and health promotion background, in conjunction with her personal experience managing her own rheumatoid arthritis and osteoporosis, has made her a strong advocate for skeletal medical issues. Gwen co-founded a chapter of the Rheumatology Nurses Society and is in constant demand as a conference and workshop presenter.

John Wade, MD, FRCPC

John is a leading Canadian rheumatologist. He is the Medical Director for Artus Health Centre in Vancouver, British Columbia and is a Clinical Associate Professor in Rheumatology at the University of British Columbia. He completed his medical studies at the University of British Columbia and Harvard Medical School. His clinical practice is focused on optimizing quality of life for patients with joint and bone diseases. He believes that outstanding clinical assessment combined with proper medication continue to alter the lives of patients for the better. Co-author of the first and subsequent editions of *The Osteoporosis Book*, John is active in osteoporosis advances and is a respected leader in continuing medical education.

www.ingramcontent.com/pod-product-compliance
Lightning Source LLC
Chambersburg PA
CBHW050502290526
45786CB00006B/2407